HACKING HEALTH

ADVANCE PRAISE FOR THE BOOK

'एक एथलिट के रूप में मुझे ये एहसास हो गया है की अल स्वस्थ जीवन व्यवस्था अच्छे परफॉरमेंस के लिये ज़रूरी है। मेरे स्वस्थ रहने की कमीटमेंट सिर्फ़ स्ट्रेंथ, मोबिलिटी और फ्लेक्सिबिलिटी की ट्रेनिंग ही नहीं, पर मानसिक ध्यान, रिकवरी और नींद भी है। हैकिंग हेल्थ अल स्वस्थ दिमाग़ एयर स्वस्थ शरीर के सभी रहस्यों को सुलझाता है।

न्यूट्रीशन और फिटनेस से लेकर मैडिटेशन और मेंटल हेल्थ तक, ये कितने हर मुद्दे को ध्यान में रख कर लिखी गई है। प्राचीन ज्ञान के साथ साथ ये कितने मॉडर्न साइंस को भी अपनाती है। आज की दुनिया में लोग अक्सर अपने स्वास्थ्य और शरीर का ध्यान रखना भूल जाते हैं, लेकिन ये दोनों चीज़ें जीवन में सबसे ज़्यादा महत्वपूर्ण हैं। मुकेश जी ने ही किताब में अपने अनुभवों और दुर्घटनाओं को सावधानी से समझकर अपने रिसर्च में अपनाया है। हैकिंग हेल्थ स्वास्थ के विषय पर एक बेहतरीन किताब है।'—नीरज चोपड़ा, ओलंपिक चैंपियन

'As an athlete, I have come to realize that a healthy lifestyle is the foundation for high performance. My commitment to staying healthy is not just about training for strength, mobility, and flexibility, but also about mental focus, recovery, and sleep. *Hacking Health* uncovers all these, and more, secrets to a healthy mind and a healthy body.

From nutrition and fitness to meditation and mental health, the book takes a truly holistic approach, drawing on ancient knowledge as well as modern science. In today's world, people often forget to keep a check on their health and body, but it really is the most important thing. Combining Mukesh's adventures (and misadventures) with meticulous research, *Hacking Health* is the definitive guide on the subject.'—Neeraj Chopra, Olympic champion

'Weaving together history and science, anecdotes and tips, *Hacking Health* takes us on a fascinating journey through the world of health. Mukesh has created a tool kit that can help every reader begin their own health journey.'—N. Chandrasekaran, Chairperson of the Tata Group

'In *Hacking Health*, Mukesh deftly blends history and science with anecdotes and practical tips to give us a one-of-a-kind guide. He invites the reader to delve into everything from fitness and food to sleep and meditation, in pursuit of their healthiest life.'—Shwetambari Shetty, Fitness expert at cult.fit, founder of Tribe Fitness

'*Hacking Health* is extraordinary in the breadth and depth of its scope, making it a practical and modern guide to a healthy lifestyle.' —Rishabh Telang, Strength and nutrition coach, founder of Cult Gyms

HACKING HEALTH

THE ONLY BOOK YOU'LL EVER NEED TO LIVE YOUR HEALTHIEST LIFE

MUKESH BANSAL

PENGUIN
VIKING
An imprint of Penguin Random House

VIKING

USA | Canada | UK | Ireland | Australia
New Zealand | India | South Africa | China

Viking is part of the Penguin Random House group of companies
whose addresses can be found at global.penguinrandomhouse.com

Published by Penguin Random House India Pvt. Ltd
4th Floor, Capital Tower 1, MG Road,
Gurugram 122 002, Haryana, India

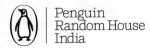

Penguin
Random House
India

First published in Viking by Penguin Random House India 2023

ISBN 9780670097135

Typeset in Minion Pro by Manipal Technologies Limited, Manipal
Printed at Thomson Press India Ltd, New Delhi

www.penguin.co.in

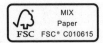

The Live Love Laugh Foundation (LLL) was founded in 2015 by actor Deepika Padukone, to give hope to every person experiencing stress, anxiety and depression. LLL focuses on increasing mental health awareness, reducing stigma related to mental illness and providing credible resources. The organization combines its expertise with partnerships and collaborations to implement outreach programs across the country.

In India, one in seven people struggles with mental illness. Many do not or cannot seek help due to the lack of awareness and stigma associated with mental illness. The modern world can be stressful and isolating and I truly believe that now, more than ever, we need to engage in meaningful conversations about mental health.

I have been inspired by LLL's efforts at the grassroots level— reaching out to students at schools and vulnerable populations in rural areas—as well as its commitment to rigorous research and capacity-building. I have chosen to donate all proceeds from this book to The Live Love Laugh Foundation towards supporting their impact initiatives in both rural and urban parts of India. If you would like to seek mental health support, learn more about the foundation or make a donation, head to www. thelivelovelaughfoundation.org or scan the QR code below.

DISCLAIMER

Before we begin, I'd like to emphasize that I am not a medical professional, and no part of this book is intended to be read as medical advice. I am passionate about health and have read extensively on the subject, while experimenting with my own routines. Drawing on all of this, I have attempted to distil the core principles in the field of health for you, the reader.

I hope this book can offer you a glimpse into the fascinating history of health and offer you tips to take your health into your own hands. However, if you intend to start a new dietary, fitness, or health regimen, take a supplement, or change a lifestyle habit, you should always consult a medical expert before doing so.

IT'S ALWAYS TEAMWORK!

I get to be the author of this book, but the truth is, I have countless people to thank who have made this book possible. While the opinions expressed are mine and I take responsibility for any omissions or mistakes, the book wouldn't have been possible without contributions from the folks mentioned below.

I must start with Aneesha Bangera, who probably read everything that was ever published on the topic of health and drove comprehensive research and analysis that forms the basis of much of the core material in the book.

I am grateful to Rishabh Telang, Ritesh Telang, Aruna Prasad, Pooja Naik, Santhosh J., Divya Rolla, Preksha Parmar, Anu Saraogi, Dr Shyam Bhat and Shwetambari Shetty for helping research, review and provide a lot of useful content and stories that have made the book simpler and easier to read.

The wonderful people at Penguin India have supported and believed in this book right from the start, and for that I am very grateful. A special thanks to my editors Manasi Subramaniam and

Shreya Punj for their attention to detail and thoughtful feedback which have made this a better book.

It has been a privilege working at CULT for the last six years as I have got to work with an amazing team of trainers, coaches, therapists and nutritionists to learn about the intricacies of health and its practical implementation.

CULT has now served millions of people who have gone on to achieve dramatic transformations, losing tens of kilograms of weight, run marathons, climb mountains and even represent India in various sports. Their stories are inspiring and their inputs not only help make CULT a better product, but they have also helped validate many of the concepts presented in this book. I can't be thankful enough.

CONTENTS

PART 3: TACKLING HEALTH GOALS

PART 4: THE FUTURE

FOREWORD
N. CHANDRASEKARAN

The subject of health is the most important subject for all. Everyone starts paying attention to health at some point in their lives, most a little later than they should. The topic of health encompasses mind, body, diet and exercise. It is really a whole-body ecosystem, and each person is distinct in terms of heredity as well as lifestyle circumstance.

Weaving together history and science, anecdotes and tips, *Hacking Health* takes us on a fascinating journey through the world of health. The book deftly combines ancient wisdom with cutting-edge science and tools that are the future of health. It separates truth from myth and demystifies what can be a complex and confusing subject. With refreshing honesty, Mukesh also gives us a glimpse into the ups and downs of his own health journey. Based on his experiences and experiments with everything from diet and fasting to sleep and tracking devices, he has created a road map and a tool kit that can help every reader begin their own health journey. Mukesh also offers simple rules to guide healthier choices and habits for better long-term health.

As a marathon runner, I experience the difference a morning run can make to my day. Beyond the more obvious physical health benefits of cardio exercise, it leaves my mind feeling fresh. As a result, I have more energy and am more productive at work and feel more positive about everything I do. While I started with running, my relationship with fitness has deepened over the years. In the process, I have incorporated various forms of fitness from strength, flexibility to meditation. I have also experienced the journey of understanding the role of food in our wellbeing. Good health enables us to lead a good life, develop a sense of composure and build deeper relationships.

Hacking Health is truly a timely book. We are emerging from the COVID-19 pandemic that affected the entire globe—a crisis that put immense pressure on our health care systems. However, we are also living in a remarkable time of science and progress—technology is transforming every system of our life and health is no exception. *Hacking Health* digs into some of these exciting developments, particularly those happening in the field of ageing and longevity. I share Mukesh's excitement at the prospect of witnessing the future of health unfold before our eyes, translating into a much longer health span for humanity.

I know Mukesh is passionate about performance and productivity and he backs himself with rigorous research, deliberate practice and a scientific approach. Mukesh gives us an informative yet accessible book that is a pleasure to read.

23 November 2022

INTRODUCTION

One summer's day in May 2007, I walked into an emergency room in San Mateo, California, at five in the morning. I hadn't slept in over forty-eight hours and had a throbbing headache as well as an inability to look directly into light. I had tried to shrug this all off as jet lag since I had been travelling back and forth between India and the US every month during the early days of Myntra. However, it soon became too painful to endure and I had no choice but to head to emergency. So, I walked in, zombie-like, and the moment the resident doctor saw me, she knew something was quite seriously wrong. On a hunch, she told me that she wanted to do a spinal tap, in which a syringe is inserted into the spinal cord, to extract fluid for testing. I, of course, had no idea what she was thinking then, and was just happy to be in the hospital and be attended to. After my spinal tap, the sample was shipped off to the lab and I was put on painkillers.

Another doctor woke me up that afternoon with a worried look. He said my sample had tested positive for meningitis, an infection of the brain and spine that can be quite deadly, depending on the strain. I would need to be completely quarantined for a few days until the doctors understood what type of meningitis they were dealing with. Confused and delirious, I started making frantic calls to close family and friends to let them know what was going on. I even called my Myntra co-founder in the middle of the night, blathering on about not knowing whether I would make it! Images and memories flashed through my mind in rapid succession most importantly—the face of my two-year-old daughter, who I had hardly seen over the previous six months as I had been spending most of that time in India, trying to bootstrap Myntra.

Within thirty minutes, I was strapped to a gurney and shipped off to the neurology ward of another hospital in an ambulance, its siren blaring as it glided surprisingly seamlessly through the otherwise notorious traffic of the Bay Area. I was put on an even stronger painkiller and antiviral medication, and I slept through the next two days as I waited for more reports. The access to my room was limited, and anyone coming in to deliver food or medicine had to be covered from head to toe—an image that continually reinforced the fear that I was carrying something catastrophic inside my brain. Finally, the lab confirmed that it was indeed meningitis, but of the viral variety, which is much easier to deal with than the more deadly bacterial strain. I continued my antiviral medication and was discharged from the hospital a few days later, fully cleared of the viral infection but extremely weak and fatigued. This horrendous ordeal, capping off a long run of falling sick nearly every month over the previous six months, made me think very seriously about giving up entrepreneurship, but I managed to stay in the game.

This experience was the new start of my health journey, as I really wanted to understand what had happened to me and how I could stop it from happening again. I used to think of myself as quite fit and healthy, as I had always played sports and had been pursuing my interest in body building for several years. It is only much later that I realized what a narrow understanding of health this was. It struck me that all the factors that go into health are much more nuanced and fascinating than I'd ever thought. This journey, that started with a harrowing experience in an emergency room fifteen years ago, continues. Over this time, I have read numerous books, experimented with all kinds of diets and fitness regimens and subjected myself to almost every test that I could get my hands on. At some point along the way, I understood that what had happened to me was related to immunity.

Our immune system is an extraordinarily sophisticated one that keeps us safe from pathogens. At times though, it can get compromised due to bad lifestyle choices, such as a lack of sleep, excessive stress, jet lag, poor food habits, recurring infections and a lack of exercise. I had fallen into almost all of these poor habits in the six months prior to my hospitalization, as I was spending three weeks in India and one in the US every single month—eating out, hardly getting any sleep on a twenty-four-hour flight as I hopped between time zones and experiencing the usual stress of building an early-stage company. A compromised immune system can affect the blood–brain barrier that filters out harmful pathogens from entering the brain. In my case, the immune system was clearly so depleted that the virus was able to enter and incubate in the brain, leading to that bout of meningitis and triggering some real soul-searching.

Having studied health for the last fifteen years, practiced varied regimens, and been engaged in the business of keeping people healthy through Cure.Fit over the last six years, my understanding of the field has dramatically improved. What I now understand is that it is both extremely simple and extraordinarily complicated. There are no more than a few simple rules that, if followed diligently, can lead to very good long-term health. But if you want to understand the underlying science and how we got to where we are now, it is a fascinating story that continues to evolve. In this book I have tried to cover both the simple advice for a healthy lifestyle and the science that makes us believe it is so. In fact, I believe that a healthy lifestyle can be boiled down to the following: Sleep more, Eat less and always Move. That's it. If you can do these three things assiduously, you don't need this book. But if you would like to understand why this works, read on! I couldn't be more excited about sharing the amazing story of health with you.

* * *

Most of us service our cars without fail every six months, using the best possible fuel to make them run smoothly. When it comes to our own annual health checks and diets, however, we often aren't so careful. Our bodies are infinitely more complex than cars and require far more care if we want to get the best mileage out of them. Alas, we often decide to put effort into looking after our bodies only when something breaks down. Someone who lives life proudly declaring their 'sweet tooth', for example, suddenly discovers the willpower to give up sugar only when confronted with a grim diagnosis of diabetes.

Thankfully, the discourse on health has become more mainstream in the last few decades. Despite the advances in our understanding and awareness of good health, however, we are also driven in multiple conflicting directions that make the pursuit of health even more challenging and confusing.

One of the things that has had a significant harmful impact on health is the modern middle-class lifestyle; one that is being pursued with more vigour than ever. Falling prices, aspirational imagery and ubiquitous access fuel this, roping in unsuspecting victims by the million every year. One element of this lifestyle is the vast array of packaged snacks and sugary drinks that is advertised to us in the name of 'happiness', leading to record levels of sugar consumption from a very early age. A large number of packaged snacks are loaded with high fructose corn syrup, a cheaper sugar substitute, that wreaks havoc on our sugar regulation mechanism and turbo-charges the weight gain processes. Another element of modern life is the ever increasing consumption of content in the guise of enriching our lives, all while we become more and more sedentary. When we called those glued to their television sets in the 1980s and 1990s 'couch potatoes', we really had no idea about what was to come! In this era of live streaming, offered virtually free so that our attention can be constantly mined, people are consuming content like never before—at home, at the office, while commuting, while working out. As if this was not enough, real-time social media on smartphones has turned most of us into zombies, going about the world tapping our fingers on the screens of shiny devices. Whether we're at the dinner table with family, out with friends, in a work meeting or walking on the pavement, our true attention is commanded by the little device in our hands.

So here we are, feeding ourselves endless sugary and salty snacks, constantly watching our screens while on a social media frenzy, and the situation is getting more dire every day. No age group is immune to this modern hysteria. Whether it is children being enticed with shiny toys served alongside fried snacks as they gaze at their iPads, or their parents glued to their mobile phones working like human routers all day to flood WhatsApp groups with everything from fake news to tasteless jokes—everyone is producing and consuming content at ever accelerating rates. We were warned of Big Brother watching our every move and people being controlled like zombies, but did we ever imagine it would largely be self-inflicted?

Don't get me wrong. This is not a rant against technology. I am a computer science engineer and a huge proponent of technology, which I think makes our lives better in innumerable ways. It just happens to be a tool that can be used for immense good but can also be exploited on a massive scale to cause damage—to the environment and human health. One could argue that due to lax regulations, many corporations, whose sole motive is to maximize profits, have benefitted hugely from feeding us mass-produced cheap snacks, bringing us endless content and capturing our attention via social media. Even though there is now incontrovertible evidence pointing to the harmful effects of all three, regulations and awareness are yet to catch up. There is no doubt that the coming decade will see more and more mainstream recognition of the harmful health impacts of these industries and technologies. Until then, however, billions must pay the cost, being sucked in by the temptation of momentary pleasure which is very hard to resist and very easy to get addicted to. Just as candy is scientifically engineered to get us hooked, the content we're being fed is also carefully designed by some of the brightest minds of our generation. Who would have thought that a computer science PhD from an Ivy League school would be the surest path to building tools that would wreak havoc on the health of millions of people?

But it's not all bad and there is still plenty of cause for optimism. Just as awareness about the environment has been increasing for many decades, there has been a surge in health awareness recently. Health is one of the most searched topics online. Afflicted by obesity, depression, and all kinds of lifestyle diseases, people are increasingly seeking information on health. Most hope for a miracle remedy for problems that are caused by years or even decades of neglect. Unfortunately, there are no quick fixes, but there is a lot of robust science that one can rely on to craft a journey towards a healthier lifestyle, even reversing the harm that poor choices in the past have caused. More awareness is certainly a good starting point, and whether one starts with walking ten thousand steps a day, eating more spinach or shunning packaged snacks—any start is a good one.

The fact that you have picked up this book is a sign that something in your life has inspired you to learn more about health and maybe do something about it. If the number of websites and blogs devoted to health and the popularity of health books are anything to go by, there is a mass awareness movement afoot that will hopefully make the pursuit of good health easy.

But therein lies a problem as well. With hundreds of health books published each year, many of which espouse the miraculous benefits of a chosen diet, superfood or practice, there is also utter confusion. Sometimes it seems easier not to do anything at all than to even try to figure it out. Are saturated fats good for us or are they the devil? Is coffee good for us? In fact, could we make up our minds about coffee once and for all, please? The continuous back and forth of theories within the field of health science, alongside a fair share of pseudoscience, makes it hard for anyone who is trying to embark on a health journey. If there seems to be no consensus on what's good for health and what isn't, where does one even begin? This is why it's so easy to fall into the trap of new fad diets and superfood trends, pursuing each as if it were a panacea for every affliction. Of course, one usually reaches a stage of disillusionment, falling back even harder than before on their earlier habits and lifestyle, none the wiser after their short-lived affair with health.

But if one parses through all the health literature, both ancient and modern, stays on the side of peer-reviewed science and marries the evidence with a bit of folk wisdom that has stood the test of time, it is not actually as difficult as it seems to tease out certain fundamental principles. Even though the principles might be simple, at no point in this book will I argue that the pursuit of a healthy lifestyle is easy. If you are willing to give up your modern city life to go live in the mountains like a monk, it may be easy (depending on your definition of easy), but otherwise, on most days, it will seem like an uphill battle, at least until a few fundamental changes become second nature.

It is interesting that we have dubbed a variety of malaises 'lifestyle diseases' with what seems like a bit of fatalism baked into the phrase. Just as night follows day, we seem to have come to terms with the idea that the lifestyle we have chosen will lead to lifestyle diseases. As much as 25 per cent of our planet suffers from lifestyle diseases and over 50 per cent of the population will suffer from these at some stage in their lives. For highly debilitating diseases that take away decades of vitality and productivity, the idea of a 'lifestyle disease' seems a convenient excuse that masks our inability or unwillingness to change the way we live. There is absolutely no evidence to prove that lifestyle diseases are inevitable. They are nothing but a by-product of a social–industrial complex that harnesses humans first as consumption machines, which inevitably leads to a decline in health, and then as consumers of extremely expensive and lifetime (how convenient!) medications to help manage these diseases. There is no doubt that a time will come when people look back at this century with more than a little curiosity at how oddly we chose to live our lives.

One of the most profound impacts of technology is that we now have the entire world's knowledge at our fingertips. Although with just a little effort, we can figure out where mainstream science stands on the topic of health and what is being pursued at the cutting edge, it still might be difficult to parse fads from truth.

This is what I intend to do through this book. Health has been a topic of interest for me over the last two decades and I have pursued every possible fad diet, workout regimen and new age supplement to see how these affect me. I have seen what was supposedly bad for us a decade ago now being promoted as a health food. I have read hundreds of books and research papers on the topic and tried a variety of things myself to develop a deeper understanding. I now believe that the pursuit of a healthy lifestyle is actually based on a few simple principles. If I had to summarize the key tenets of a healthy lifestyle as simply as I could, it would be as follows:

1. Get seven to eight hours of sleep every night
2. Be physically active everyday, it doesn't matter how
3. Eat locally sourced raw and cooked food
4. Cultivate mindfulness
5. Pursue goals that have meaning for you
6. Nurture healthy relationships

The challenge, however, is not in knowing what leads to a healthy lifestyle, but in how to actually incorporate these elements in your everyday life. The biggest obstacle to good health is that it is not like a flu shot that you need to get just once a year. The pursuit of good health requires making healthy choices almost every day, year after year, and this is why it is challenging. You may have all the best intentions to get a full night's sleep, but then you find yourself riveted to a thrilling show or out at a party where you don't want to be called the party pooper. Something within you reminds you that 'you live only once' and you give in to this feeling, hoping to fully enjoy the moment, never mind that all your plans for the next day are already bust. Or you started with a resolve to avoid all sugar this week. And then one day nothing seems to be in order at work. As you walk out of a stressful meeting, you see a freshly baked brownie on the office kitchen counter and without even noticing it, you devour two, triggering a chain reaction of guilt even before the brownie has settled in. This is how most health journeys go. Death by a thousand cuts.

So, what gives? If on one hand a healthy lifestyle is just about getting a few things right, why is it still next to impossible? I don't think there are any easy answers or magic pills. Good health boils down to having the right information and ideas, translating them into creating an environment with fewer temptations, and then cultivating habits that turn new behaviours to autopilot so that we make the right choices without even thinking about them. For example, packing a wholesome home-cooked meal before you go to work all but rules out the possibility of unhealthy bingeing during lunch hour. Of course, creating habits is far from easy, which is why we often give up before something has firmly become a part of our routine. On some days, the quick fixes and short-term gains seem so much simpler and more satisfying than buckling in for the long haul. This is normal human behaviour, so instead of constantly battling against ourselves, the best way to live a healthier lifestyle is to make choices that are sustainable, easy to incorporate into our daily life and bring us joy.

My goal in this book is to deconstruct health into its building blocks, to review the science, history and relevant studies and to boil it all down to easy choices that you can incorporate into your daily routine. You may agree with some of the viewpoints and may want to challenge others, which is absolutely fine as there are many areas in health where we still don't have very robust science, leaving things open to cultural and personal interpretation. You can also choose to experiment with a few ideas, see how you feel when you try them out and decide if they work for you or not.

Take **fitness** as an example. Unless you have a very specific athletic or aesthetic goal, good health requires you to be physically active in any way you like. Over the last two decades, I have done everything from serious weightlifting to middle distance running to playing sports to practising yoga to just taking long walks and I think each of these, as well as every other activity that involves movement of the body, are all legitimate ways to stay healthy.

From fitness we shift to **food**, where things get terribly interesting but also terribly confusing. The simple job of providing our bodies with enough nutrient-rich calories to run has become incredibly complex, with dozens of fad diets and food trends to choose from. But no matter what diet you choose to follow, it is amply clear that there is no one-stop magic solution that will work for everyone. Whatever you choose, your body will give you feedback if you only stop and listen. Good food makes you feel alive and vibrant while unhealthy food makes you feel dull and lethargic.

While food and fitness get an inordinate amount of attention in all health discussions, **sleep** might be one of the most fundamental pillars. There is absolutely no pursuit of good health without good sleep, and yet most people approach it as a necessary evil and try to get by on as little sleep as possible. It is only in very recent times that we have started to chip away at the mystery of sleep and now understand the profound processes that our brain undergoes while we sleep, which have a huge impact on every aspect of our health.

It is no wonder then, that there is no elixir like a good night's sleep for true vitality.

One of the most exciting recent contributions of health science is the reawakening of focus on **mindfulness** and **meditation**. This is a perfect example of life coming full circle. In every ancient religious practice, there has always been a great deal of emphasis on developing the habit of focusing one's attention on something, developing detached attachment and cultivating more awareness. Now, science tells us that even a few minutes of meditation every day has a profound impact on our brains, and that pursuing mindfulness imparts meaning to what we do, leading to a feeling of overall happiness.

The COVID-19 pandemic has highlighted issues of immunity—and how to boost it—more than ever before, exposing the perils of living in crowded and polluted metropolises. Falling sick every few months doesn't have to be the norm, however, with lifestyle interventions that can improve productivity and long-term health.

Another scourge of modern living is the rapid rise of mental illnesses, from anxiety to depression, that take a silent toll on us. Unfortunately, there is still a lot of stigma attached to these in India and these diseases often go undiagnosed for years. Better awareness, access to therapy and medication and lifestyle changes can help us better care for our mental health.

An epidemic that seems to have no limit is obesity, which is highly correlated with chronic long-term health issues. In this book, we attempt to delve into the mechanism at work in those with obesity, understanding how we can make real change rather than offer quick fixes that don't last.

One of the very significant developments in the field of health is how much we are able to measure what is going on with our bodies. Instead of trying to intuit how we feel at a particular time, we can know exactly what is going on with our health using a multitude of wearable devices that, if we want, will track our health 24X7. We can go one step further and get genetic testing done to analyse our ancestral blueprint which can alert us to dangers that lurk in our DNA and what we can do to avert potential pitfalls. We are moving towards a world where health will cease to be some kind of black box where mysterious things happen on their own. Instead, we will have more of a dashboard like that of a car, where we have a dedicated gauge for each function and we can know exactly what is working, what isn't or what needs fine tuning.

While we will talk about all the perils of our modern lifestyle and the devastating effect it is having on our health, I would be amiss if I don't simultaneously talk about all the exciting work that is going on at the cutting edge of health, where credible scientists are working on solving the problem of ageing itself. Even though people have fantasized about the elixir of youth since ancient times and there are mythological stories galore about the eternal fountain of youth, these were never more than flights of fancy. But in the last few decades, we have been able to look much deeper into the science of ageing, questioning whether ageing as we now know it is inevitable at all.

That lays the outline of what we will cover in this book. I like to think of it as a whirlwind tour of the world of health with a focus on what you can do right now to boost your health. We will demystify many myths and acknowledge some of the ancient wisdom, which is still as cutting-edge as it was when first conceived.

Health is a true enabler for a life of productivity and meaning and it is well within our reach. We are a unique generation in the sense that we are simultaneously cursed with more health issues than any generation before us but also armed with more tools and understanding than anyone ever before. It is my endeavour to help you navigate the seemingly complex world of health, highlight some very simple principles and equip you with the tools to begin your own journey towards a life filled with vitality and good health.

To good health. Let's begin!

PART 1

FUNDAMENTALS OF GOOD HEALTH

1

HEALTH RULES

Eat food, not too much, mostly plants.—Michael Pollan

For as long as humans have had to deal with disease and death, they have been interested in better health. We have paid attention to our health by making conscious lifestyle choices, or by encoding these in rituals, behaviours and products. For example, iodine is almost universally added to table salt to ensure that our bodies receive this vital mineral, without us having to worry about supplementation. As human societies evolved, they observed patterns that were beneficial for good health and continued to codify these, teaching the next generation and sometimes even incorporating them in sacred commandments. Sometimes, people got it right, while at others, blind faith along with the body's susceptibility to the placebo effect worked too.

Hippocrates, known as the Father of Medicine, famously wrote, 'Let food be thy medicine', something he practiced with every patient—prescribing a change in diet to treat illnesses. It seems that the idea of food as medicine is almost as old as medicine itself.

For most of ancient history, health rules were the outcome of trial and error. People would adopt a new plan and observe their reaction to it. If it worked, it would become part of a toolkit for better health. For example, it would have been pretty obvious that people who didn't get enough sleep would feel listless the next day. This is possibly why good sleep has been universally promoted across all cultures.

As our understanding of health grew exponentially through rigorous scientific studies, so did a giant industry selling a 'get rich quick' equivalent of products for health. From magical superfoods to miracle pills and powders that claim to instantly teleport you to the promised land of blissful health and harmony, this industry thrives on our eternal quest for better health. There is no doubt that much of the marketing in this industry relies on limited or questionable science and exaggerated results, not to mention the vested interests of powerful lobbies. For example, the sugar lobby is responsible for nearly banning saturated fat, despite no concrete evidence against it. In fact, most mainstream nutrition establishments now deem saturated fat a highly essential ingredient for good health. I should have never given up ghee, something that I grew up eating and loving, until the low-fat lobby stripped all the joy out of it. Darn it!

If we take a step back and survey everything that we now know about the pursuit of good health, certain patterns emerge which form the backbone of almost all health advice. These are time-tested insights, deeply ingrained in ancient culture and validated by modern science. If you understand these rules and incorporate some of them in your life, you will see more lasting change than when you follow some fad diet or popular workout until you get bored and move on to the next one. These rules will also help you evaluate new health advice, helping you gauge if it is based on the fundamentals of health, or on some fly-by-night theories and products. Let's dive in and explore the fundamental rules for good health.

RULE 1: USE IT OR LOSE IT

Until a century ago, one of the most vexing problems faced by all life on this planet was that of energy, which is why the bodies of all living organisms evolved to be energy efficient. It is precisely for this reason that the body doesn't tolerate what it sees as a useless part, eventually dissolving it and using it for energy. You see this in action when you have a cast on for a fracture. When the cast is removed, the limb is noticeably thinner. Seeing that the muscles were not being used, your body literally digested them for calories. Being self-consumed takes on a whole different meaning sometimes!

The same thing happens in reverse when you exercise a particular muscle—the more you work it, the more it responds by growing and strengthening.

Many of us are fairly physically active until high school or college, and then our lives turn so sedentary that we can barely run 100 m without having to stop to catch our breath. During those years of inactivity, the body sheds the muscular endurance and flexibility it had when it was in its prime. However, barring a small age tax, you can get back into shape with conditioning over a period of time. Your body is incredibly smart and very frugal— letting go of capabilities that aren't being used, but also responding powerfully and quickly to training.

So, this is the first rule on the route to better health. If you want stronger calf muscles or bigger biceps, you have to train and, under the right conditions, your body will build them. Similarly, what you don't use will wither away, whether it is a physical ability or a mental faculty. That's it, use it, or lose it. None of this happens overnight, but the effects add up over the months and years. As you start to think about your health, you need to pay attention to what you spend most of your time doing. What you do every day is what your body will become.

HEALTH HACK #1: Move

Our bodies are designed for movement, so moving is good for health. Find ways to move every day, whether by cycling into work, or walking to the grocery store and hauling your shopping back rather than ordering online. To make movement a habit, sign up for a fitness class to make yourself more accountable.

RULE 2: BACK TO THE BASICS

Our ancestors spent most of the last 2,00,000 years as hunter–gatherers, right up until the dawn of agriculture about 10,000 years ago.

Most human tribes traditionally lived in groups of 150 people or fewer, living off the natural resources in their area, walking several kilometres every day in search of tubers, fruits and edible plants, and occasionally hunting animals. Whenever a population increased beyond the number that local resources could support, groups would split, with one going off to find a new habitat.[1]

Around 10,000 years ago, with the global climate warming up, our species' growing brains discovered a more efficient way to create surplus energy through agriculture. People began to settle down in larger groups, delegating farming work to a few, while the surplus food ensured others could indulge in different activities.

This left our lifestyles dramatically altered—more so after the industrial revolution in the seventeenth century. All of a sudden, we had no need to do any manual labour or wander around, as our work was taken over by machines driven by oil and electricity. The human lifestyle has become sedentary, but our bodies are yet to catch up. Lifestyle diseases—a relatively new term—are basically diseases of too little activity, too much food and too much processed food, unlike what our ancestors ate.

This is the second rule of pursuing good health. The more our everyday lifestyles can mimic those of our hunter–gatherer ancestors, the better off we are. This means walking a lot, eating a large variety of seasonal foods (often raw), spending time in nature and sometimes just not doing anything but soaking in the wonderful world around us, as opposed sitting hunched over our desks. Our ancestors were not having to resort to munching salty packages snacks or downing sodas, while working all day, with their eyes glued to a screen, and there is no doubt we won't gain very much by doing so.

RULE 3: EAT LESS

It turns out that from ancient ascetics to modern nutrition scientists, one thing everyone agrees on are the immense benefits of calorie restriction. There are studies that show an increase of up to 50 per cent in the lifespan of lab rats on severely calorie restricted diets.[2] Reducing food intake reduces oxidative burden and damage to DNA, keeping animals in a biologically younger state. There are no long-term scientific studies involving long term calorie restriction in humans, but there is plenty of anecdotal evidence showing that it does your body a world of good.

If we go back to contemplating the lives of our hunter–gatherer ancestors in the wild, we realize that three meals a day were never guaranteed. You had to go out in search of food and some days you found something to eat, while on others you didn't. This is why our bodies have become good at storing excess calories as fat to be used for energy when food supply is running low.

It is no wonder that every major religion in the world has advocated some kind of periodic fasting. There are stories of yogis being able to go without food for days or even weeks, and now we know scientifically that while we can't survive more than a few days without water, or go without sleep for a week, we can survive without food for as long as a month! Our bodies can do without food for an extended period of time, no matter how desperately snack food companies want us to keep snacking.

As the science of nutrition has improved in the last few decades, the numerous benefits of fasting are becoming more and more evident. People may prescribe different methods for intermittent fasting ranging from fourteen hours to forty-eight hours, but in truth it doesn't really matter. If you can manage to skip a meal or two occasionally your body will thank you for it and your long-term health will reflect it.

HEALTH HACK #2: Continuous Glucose Monitoring

A continuous glucose monitoring (CGM) device is a nifty gadget to track blood sugar levels through the day and night. Either inserted beneath the skin of the stomach or worn attached to the arm, it transmits information to a monitor that displays glucose levels every five to fifteen minutes.

Rule 4: Just Move

Our bodies were designed for regular movement. Our ancestors walked, ran, climbed, swam and hunted, and only rarely spent time sitting in one position. They left the African savannah a few hundred thousand years ago and, without any technology or protection, ended up reaching every last corner of the Earth, adapting themselves to the coldest and hottest regions, crossing mountains and oceans, surviving ice ages and droughts, outsmarting fearsome creatures and overcoming just about every obstacle nature threw their way. The only thing that they didn't do was sit still in front of a screen all day.

Every part of our bodies is designed for movement. Our feet have the largest number of intricate muscles that perform marvellous feats of engineering, not only allowing us to balance on two legs, but enabling us to walk, run, jump and even stand on one leg.

When we are moving, our hearts beat faster, pumping more blood to our extremities; we engage our brains more as we come across new inputs, and we exercise most of our muscles, which we know work on the 'use it or lose it' principle. There is no part of our evolutionary history that required us to sit on our haunches all day long (although sitting directly on the floor is still better than on a chair, as this position stretches all our muscles).

Movement is so critical for both our minds and bodies that it almost doesn't matter how you do it. Sure, you can have a very fancy training routine for specific aesthetic or performance goals, but don't underestimate the positive impact of just standing up and walking.

Rule 5: Be Still

All of humanity's problems stem from man's inability to sit quietly in a room alone. —Blaise Pascal

While movement is essential for good health, moments of stillness are just as important for the body and the mind. Wise people of all ages and cultures have practiced long bouts of silence and meditation to get in touch with their inner voices and to tease out deeper wisdom from the universe. A core tenet of Zen Buddhism is contemplation in stillness. In ancient Yogic traditions, meditation is considered the most important aspect of the journey to self-realization, leading to an appreciation of greater truths. In Jainism, monks are expected to observe periods of silence lasting weeks, while in Vipassana meditation, participants disconnect from all interactions and observe complete silence for ten days, directing all attention inward.

Compare this to our modern lives in which we spend our time shuttling from one interruption to another. Social media and mobile phones take distraction to another level altogether, filling us with the irresistible urge to reach into our pockets to check the next 'like' or to respond to the ping of a new email as soon as it arrives. In this way, we can go for hours or even days in a zombie-like trance, barely noticing what's going on around us. Sean Parker, himself an early backer of Facebook, has warned that social media is highly addictive and especially harmful to children who are particularly vulnerable during cognitive development.[3]

The mind plays a vital role in good health and without a fresh, energetic and engaged mind, it is difficult to feel healthy or make healthy choices. A tired or distracted mind is far more likely to give in to temptation. Have you ever noticed how quickly a gigantic bag of popcorn disappears while you're binge watching your favourite TV show?

A healthy mind requires dedicated periods of stillness. You can meditate, go for a walk, journal, listen to music or just sit and daydream. You will be surprised by how alive and alert you feel, and your mind will thank you for this increasingly rare luxury that is so vital to our well-being.

Rule 6: Sleep Your Way to Good Health

For a large part of human history, sleep was a mystery, and seemed to serve no purpose beyond being a source of dreams for interpretation. Even if people felt great after a good night's rest, most would lament the colossal waste of time. After all, nobody wanted to spend a third of their lives in what was thought to be a coma-like stupor that had no benefits. And now we know that they could not have been more wrong! Sleep is one of the most critical elements of good health. If there is just one thing you could do for your health, it should be to get seven to eight hours of sleep regularly. For those with the luxury, it is even advisable to sleep for as long as your body needs, without an alarm!

Thanks to advanced brain imaging technologies, we now know that in sleep, our brains are equally as, or perhaps even more, active as when we are awake, albeit in a very different way.

At night, the brain processes everything that it experienced during the day, deciding what to transition into long term memory and what to discard. This is why good sleep is so critical for learning. During illness or injury, most recovery happens while you sleep. If you work out vigorously, it is during sleep that the muscles will be repaired to become stronger.

We now have numerous studies that link good quality sleep with good health at all levels. From boosting immunity and learning to improving mental health, from improving willpower and athletic performance to helping people live longer, sleep is that elusive miracle drug whose benefits are seemingly endless. There is no good health without good sleep. Period.

RULE 7: USING HORMESIS: CONTROLLED STRESS FOR THE BODY

Mithridates the Great, the king of Pontus, was one of the Romans' greatest foes, but while he was considered a great leader, he was plagued by the fear of being poisoned. To find ways of protecting himself, he began to dabble in toxicology, and is believed to have self-administered non-lethal doses of poisonous substances in order to protect himself from them.[4] If indeed this is true, Mithridates was inadvertently tapping into the concept of hormesis, or the ability of the body to improve itself in the face of a controlled stress environment. Nietzsche immortalized the same concept in his famous aphorism, 'What doesn't kill me makes me stronger.'[5]

The science of vaccination works on the very same principle. A vaccine hacks into the body's natural hormetic response, turning it into a powerful weapon against deadly diseases.

Wim Hof, known as the Ice Man, takes hormesis to the next level by controlling his body's response to the cold through a specific technique of breathing and cold exposure. Hof has climbed Mount Kilimanjaro in shorts, run a marathon above the Arctic Circle in bare feet and broken several records of cold exposure. Studies have since found that the method activates a part of the brain involved in pain suppression, while practitioners of the method appear to have better control of their sympathetic nervous system. Leveraging hormesis, Wim Hof has developed abilities so far believed to be beyond human grasp.

Mimicking some of the survival circuits of our evolutionary ancestors, such as fasting or restricting caloric intake, can also bring us several benefits—another example of hormesis at work.

So, if you want to make your mind and body better, you will have to expose yourself to controlled stress and then provide adequate nutrition and rest for the body to repair itself. That's how you get better. Nothing good happens while you're cocooned in a comfort zone, no matter how good you may feel in that moment!

Rule 8: Embrace the Mind-Body Connection

The mind–body dichotomy has baffled philosophers since time immemorial. Humans have long grappled with the question of whether the mind is just a manifestation of the physical construct of our brains, or something more ephemeral and universal. Truth be told, these questions are still far from being completely resolved, but according to the most sophisticated understanding of neuroscience currently, there are physical underpinnings to everything that goes on in our minds, from the most primitive cravings to the most transcendental thoughts.

One of the most profound understandings of the last fifty years is how intricately connected the mind and body are. The euphoric sense of elation after a really intense run or workout, known as the 'runner's high' and caused by an increase in the supply of dopamine, is a great example of how physical exertion affects the mind. Similarly, after a few breathing exercises or meditation, your performance on a physical task may improve considerably. It has been proven repeatedly, that visualization exercises help increase performance in sport, a decidedly physical activity.

An ancient Kurdish saying gets it right. 'The root of all health is in the brain. The trunk of it is in emotion. The branches and leaves are the body. The flower of health blooms when all parts work together.' In fact, almost all ancient medical practices, including yoga, were truly holistic in the sense that they treated the mind and body not as separate entities but as a whole.

Another very significant example of the mind–body connection is how gut health affects the brain. Every time you overeat or snack on junk food, you probably feel lethargic and even mildly depressed. Our gut has been dubbed the 'second brain' because it regulates many powerful neurotransmitters which affect how the brain feels and performs.

When looking at your health, it is important to know that you can no longer isolate the mind from the body, or vice versa, and that to improve the health of either one, you need to address both. Our bodies and minds are far too intricately connected to be treated as separate entities, and recognizing this connection is extremely important in the pursuit of health.

RULE 9: PURPOSE MATTERS . . . A LOT

Can having a meaningful life make you healthier? Several studies have shown that there is indeed a connection between a sense of purpose and a longer and healthier life. It boils down to the fact that if you have something meaningful to live for, chances are you will live longer. It is also why many retirees, who don't have a strong sense of purpose beyond their careers, tend to see a rapid decline in their health in the first decade after retirement.

Research has found that, among some groups studied, those above a certain age who report a lack of purpose or meaning in their lives are almost twice as likely to die as those who have a reason to get out of bed every morning.[6] In fact, this study concluded that purpose was a factor more closely associated with longevity than any other, including gender, race and economic background. Researchers suggest that people who have a strong purpose feel a need to live longer, and this motivates them to seek wellbeing. For example, an elderly person who is a grandparent might want to stay healthy and live longer in order to watch their grandchildren grow up. To this end, they might start engaging in some daily physical activity, or eating more nutritiously.

What this could mean for us is that by actively seeking out a purpose in our lives—whether it is family, a passion project or a deep sense of spirituality—we could be doing the right thing for our health in the long run.

HEALTH HACK #3: Community Dining

Eating meals together is something that most families did until recently, and it turns out that it's not just good for conversation, but also for health. Families that eat together tend to make healthier dietary choices, are less likely to be obese and, in general, experience more wellness and joy.

RULE 10: GET SOCIAL

The way our societies have developed in the last few decades means that many people now live several thousands of miles away from their families and their roots. While technology helps bring us together in many ways, it has also contributed to a sense of isolation. As a result, despite living in crowded metropolises, many people are essentially lonely. And science now tells us that loneliness is bad for our health.

Cultivating strong relationships with family, friends and the community can have a very powerful positive impact on our health. This might be why one of the most horrific torture methods is social isolation. Numerous studies have found that having strong social bonds is correlated with having better health and living longer.[7] People who are married, in long-term relationships or who have strong social ties with their friends seem to take better care of their health, have better access to healthcare and are more likely to seek treatment.

When researchers looked into the common traits shared by populations in the Blue Zones of the world—regions where people consistently live to ages of 100 and above—one of the most common findings was very strong local communities, with people caring for each other, celebrating together and being meaningfully involved in each other's lives.

Almost everything that we will cover in this book stems from these rules. Health doesn't need to be elusive or a mystery. The ability to stay healthy is built into our biology and our success as a species is a testament to this fact. Yes, our health might have gone a bit haywire recently but with an understanding of how health works and with simple changes, we can all pursue a much healthier lifestyle. Investing in good health now will bring benefits for decades.

In Summary

- Rule No. 1: Use It or Lose It: When it comes to the health of the body and mind, you have to use it or lose it. Staying physically and mentally active can keep you in good health.
- Rule No. 2: Back to the Basics: To boost health, try and live like our hunter–gatherer ancestors—keep moving, eat fresh, seasonal and raw, and slow down.
- Rule No. 3: Eat Less: Whether it's occasionally skipping a meal, following an intermittent fasting plan, or doing longer fasts, eating fewer calories is one of the only ways of extending health and life.
- Rule No. 4: Just Move: The human body is designed for movement, so movement is essential, especially if you are required to spend long hours sitting in front of various screens.
- Rule No. 5: Be Still: Meditation and stillness are important ways of staying in touch with the self, improving both physical and mental health.
- Rule No. 6: Sleep Your Way to Good Health: Sleep might be the key to good health—playing a role in recovery, memory and learning, immunity and making you a better version of yourself.
- Rule No. 7: Using Hormesis: Stress doesn't always have to be bad for you. Small doses of controlled stress (called hormesis), such as cold exposure or in the form of vaccines, can have great benefits.
- Rule No. 8: Embrace the Mind–Body Connection: The mind is just as important to good health as the body is, and there is wellbeing only when both are cared for.

- Rule No. 9: Purpose Matters: Having a reason to wake up every morning not only gives your life meaning but can actually improve your overall health and wellness.
- Rule No. 10: Get Social: Humans are social animals and maintaining our social networks has proven to be good for health and longevity.

2

THE STORY OF HEALTH

Fifty years ago, health was not the trendy topic it is today. Perhaps we just weren't very interested in what was considered a rather boring subject back then, but we also did not have much access to information about it beyond what we might occasionally have heard from a grandparent or doctor when we were sick. Fast forward to today, and much of the content that we are bombarded with is related to health. Hidden amid selfies on your social media feeds, work emails and TV shows, you're sure to find ads promoting the latest miracle remedy for a health problem, a list of superfoods and their magical benefits, or a self-styled health guru who offers health wisdom in the form of a detox diet or a plan to get a six-pack in six weeks (or less!). By the sounds of things, it seems like several of these 'experts' have cracked the code to good health. And yet, we still find ourselves weighed down by disease and poor health.

Fortunately, alongside a lot of somewhat questionable information, there have been rapid strides too, thanks to the relentless work of health and nutrition scientists, researchers and authentic health aficionados, or biohackers. The perspective has shifted from merely enhancing longevity to the ability to make choices to live a vibrant and fulfilling life well into old age.

Before we continue our journey, I'd like to take you on a whirlwind tour of the story of health. The evolution of the modern health narrative is fascinating, and provides context for the various choices you can make today. The entire story would take many, many books, so here, we will just look at some of the key developments that shaped the world of health as we now know it.

1. GOOD CALORIES, BAD CALORIES

A good place to start our story is with food, which nourishes us and keeps us alive. A concept that has dominated the global conversation on nutrition in the recent past is the 'calorie', a subject of much contention. We count calories, compare them, choose them, condemn them, but most of us know little about how they came to have such a significant impact on the way we eat and relate to food.

The calorie was originally a unit of heat, defined as the amount of heat required to raise the temperature of 1 g of water by 1 degree Celsius. A rather bizarre experiment conducted in 1896 by a professor at Wesleyan University, Wilbur O. Atwater, brought the calorie as we now know it into the spotlight.[1] For the study, a graduate student climbed into a calorimeter, an airtight metal chamber previously used to measure the energy created by engines and explosives. He was fed measured quantities of bread, baked beans, milk, mashed potatoes and steaks, while his energy output was measured in terms of thermal energy. As a result of this experiment, foods were assigned values in terms of calories for the first time, effectively turning eating into a study of mathematics.

The idea of calories first became a tool for the US government to achieve 'nutritional efficiency', especially when it came to feeding an industrial workforce, prisoners and school children. Restaurants in New York even listed the caloric value of dishes on their menu, alongside the recommended daily calorie intake for different walks of life! During the First World War, calories played an important role in food rationing and export.

While Atwater used his discoveries to discuss achieving physiological efficiency, it was doctor and author Lulu Hunt Peters who, in 1918, began to popularize the idea of calorie counting for weight loss. Through her weekly column and a book titled *Diet and Health: With Key to the Calories*, she advocated subtracting calories from one's diet to lose weight. At a time when skinny was 'in', her approach reduced food entirely to its constituent calories. Peters famously wrote, 'Hereafter, you are going to eat calories of food. Instead of saying one slice of bread, or a piece of pie, you will say 100 calories of bread, 350 calories of pie.'[2] After Peters, it seems, there was no looking back. Calories became the go-to measurement for anyone looking to lose, or in some cases gain, weight, based on the idea that consuming fewer calories than you expend leads to weight loss, while consuming more than you spend results in weight gain.

Both Atwater and Peters contributed to the rise of nutrition as a quantifiable science, which in some ways took food traditions out of their rich social and cultural contexts and histories.

One of the most commonly held beliefs for a long time was that a calorie is a calorie, no matter where it comes from. A 1903 ad for beer in the Washington Post went as far as claiming that a glass of their beer was almost equal in calories to a glass of milk, and therefore, was enough to 'furnish abundant energy to the human machine'.[3] In fact, Atwater did not consider green, leafy vegetables healthy—he barely considered them food—because they contained so few calories that they were not efficient sources of energy in his eyes.

One of the most significant fallouts of the calorie counting trend was the vilification of fats in the 1980s. Fat, the macronutrient, has the misfortune of sharing its name with the adjective for people who are overweight, and as a result we have always viewed it with some suspicion. In addition, being more calorie dense than the other macronutrients, it was assumed that fat was the main cause of weight gain. This led not only to the rise of processed carbohydrates in our diets, which we now know are not very high in nutritional value, but also to people choosing low-fat or fat-free products, thinking these would help them keep their weight in check. The problem, however, is that most low-fat products are high in sugars. Thinking they were making the healthy choice, people would avoid fries but make their soda large—a soda which might have had as many as ten tablespoons of sugar!

The thing about calories is that, sometimes, it's more about quality than quantity (like a lot of things in our lives!), and we will examine this in greater detail in the next chapter.

2. THE FOOD LOBBY

As much as we like to think of ourselves as the masters of our own fates, the fact is that the food lobby and the world of advertisements have had a big impact on our perceptions of what is or isn't healthy. For example, margarine, a butter substitute derived from the hydrogenation of vegetable oil, was marketed as a lighter and healthier option, and consumers lapped it up. Now, however, we know that the process of hydrogenation produces trans fats that are the most harmful type of fat. There is also an entire industry built around canned juices that may sound healthy just because they contain fruit, but are in fact loaded with preservatives and added sugars.

Few of us might know this, but the idea that breakfast is the most important meal of the day might be part of a somewhat elaborate scam designed by the food lobbies. Until the nineteenth century, in the West, the first meal of the day did not consist of any specific foods, and instead involved eating leftovers from the previous night's meal or cured meats that did not require much cooking. It was only after the rise of cereal companies like Kellogg's and other so-called breakfast food companies, that advertising began to prescribe what people ate to start their days. Kellogg's propagated the idea that light and ready-to-eat meals were better for the post-industrial revolution workforce, preventing indigestion and making life easier for working mothers. Even in India, with its diversity of wholesome and delicious breakfast foods across states, many have fallen for the trap of breakfast cereals, which are marketed as a nutritious, energy packed meal to start the day.

In addition to advertising, the food industry wields immense power, influencing much of what we read about health. A paper published in 2016 revealed that the Sugar Research Foundation of the US funded research that downplayed the role of sucrose in coronary heart disease in the 1960s and 1970s. Instead, they began popularizing the idea that fat was the main cause of heart disease. Not only did these studies fail to declare the sponsorship from the SRF, but they also turned attention away from research that had begun to show the health risks caused by added sugars.[4]

Interestingly, in the early 1990s, the term 'the French Paradox' was coined to refer to the lower rates of mortality and heart disease among the French, despite a high intake of dietary cholesterol and saturated fats. While various theories were put forward, one that caught people's imagination was that the consumption of wine in France might provide protection against the unhealthy aspects of the diet. While the theory is now considered to lack sufficient evidence, it did lead to research into the health benefits of red wine.

With the shift to mass production of processed food and quick service restaurants, there was more incentive for food producers to make food that would last longer on shelves, was cheaper to produce and was addictive. Enter the food scientists who figured out that our brains are hard-wired to release short bursts of dopamine every time we have something laden with fat, sugar or salt. All these are essential for life and are in extremely short supply in nature, so whenever we do get something with these ingredients, our mouths naturally salivate. They discovered that they could increase these elements dramatically and mix them in interesting combinations, leaving consumers salivating all day, constantly craving more. If you have ever devoured an entire bag of chips laced with generous amounts of grease and salt without even realizing where it went, you have been a victim of this industrial complex.

One of the biggest villains to emerge in this story is high fructose corn syrup (HFCS), a sugar derived from corn starch that is the most 'sugary' sugar one can produce. It is far cheaper than sugar derived from sugarcane and can be easily stored and transported. The discovery of HFCS was a breakthrough for the sugar industry, as one after another, snack and soda companies started using HFCS instead of natural sugar. The sale of HFCS soared, leading to a huge demand for corn, in turn leading to a rapid increase in the land being cultivated for corn—a story for another day, perhaps.

I have been as much a victim of the powerful food lobbies as the next person. I remember walking through the aisles of supermarkets when I lived in the US, always choosing milk with '0 per cent fat'. What I didn't realize then was that I was essentially drinking all the milk's sugars while filtering out its good fats. With better science on our side now and an awareness of the hidden interests of food lobbies, we can equip ourselves to make better dietary choices.

3. Unravelling the Mystery of Sleep

For most of our evolutionary history, sleep was merely a source of dreams and nightmares that early civilizations tried to control with chanting and medicinal plants. The eighteenth century, however, saw the beginnings of sleep science as people recognized that there was more to this night-time rest we couldn't seem to do without. The introduction of artificial lighting was perhaps the first phenomenon that altered our sleep patterns, foreshadowing the epidemic of insomnia and other sleep disorders that would plague modern humans.

The discovery of an internal or biological clock was one of the first steps towards unravelling the mystery of sleep. In 1729, French scientist Jean-Jacques d'Ortous de Mairan observed that the leaves of the *Mimosa pudica*, better known as the touch-me-not plant, opened and closed with the rising and setting of the sun. He decided to place the plant in a sealed box, where it would lie in complete darkness for twenty-four hours, to see what would happen. He went on to note that even though it had been cut off from sun exposure that indicated the passage of day, the plant continued to expand in the daytime and retract at night. This was the first demonstration that living beings had an internal mechanism to keep time, that was not entirely dependent on the movement of the sun.

Almost two hundred years later, another exciting experiment took place, in which Nathaniel Kleitman and his student, Bruce Richardson, undertook something of an adventure to see if the human circadian rhythm would descend into complete, erratic chaos, in the absence of sunlight. They attempted this by spending thirty-two days in the cold, dark and damp Mammoth Cave in Kentucky, USA, where there were no changes in light and temperature to indicate the passing of the days and nights. Using devices to measure body temperature, they also observed their waking and sleeping cycles. They discovered two significant things: one, despite the lack of light, they experienced predictable patterns of alertness and sleepiness; and two, their cycles were slightly longer than twenty-four hours. Since then, it has been determined that the human circadian rhythm runs in cycles of, on average, twenty-four hours and fifteen minutes.

It is only as recently as the mid-twentieth century that sleep scientists began to identify the different phases of sleep that we cycle through in the night, and the activity in various regions of the brain that accompany them. This finally explained why sleep is so incredibly important for health, having an impact on everything from weight management to learning and memory. Sleep science continues to be a fascinating area of research and every new revelation serves to further emphasize just how essential it is.

4. THE HUMAN GENOME

The question of how we inherit traits over generations is one that has fascinated and confounded humanity for centuries. The history of the discovery of the gene is a captivating story that perhaps began several centuries ago, but truly unfolded in the late-nineteenth and twentieth centuries.

In around 530 BC, Greek scholar Pythagoras put forward the theory that the male sperm absorbed hereditary information from the male body, travelling into the womb during intercourse, where the woman's body provided nutrition to create a child. Aristotle, however, came along to challenge Pythagoras, asking how it was, if all 'likeness' came from the father, that children often resembled their mothers or even their grandparents. Instead, he proposed the theory that from the male parent came the 'message' in the form of the sperm, while what he considered the 'female semen', or menstrual blood, contributed the 'material' that gave form to a foetus.[5]

Most theories of this time spoke of 'information', yet did not propose how the information was passed on. The answer to this came in the form of the concept of the homunculus, the idea that every sperm contains a miniscule foetus, which, when transferred to the female womb, grows into a child. For this theory of 'preformation' to work, however, every homunculus had to have an entire lineage of tiny foetuses curled up inside, what Siddhartha Mukherjee describes in his book, *The Gene: An Intimate History*, as, 'an infinite series of Russian dolls, a great chain of being that stretched all the way backward from the present to the first man, to Adam, and forward into the future.'[6] While this theory appealed to the growing Christian sentiment of the Medieval times and remained popular till the 1800s, there were still glaring holes in the story of inheritance.

It wasn't until Darwin's epic journey to the Galapagos Islands, which inspired his theory of natural selection, that the study of genetics, as we now know it, actually began.

Around the same time that Darwin published his landmark work *The Origin of Species*, an Austrian monk in Brno was breeding different strains of pea plants in the garden of his monastery.

An obsessive experimentalist, Gregor Mendel laboriously cross-pollinated variants of pea plants over almost eight years and recorded his findings meticulously. Mendel was able to demonstrate that traits were passed down from one generation to the next in indivisible units, all but laying down the conceptual underpinning of the genetic revolution that would unfold over the next hundred years.[7]

The next major breakthrough didn't occur until the 1940s, when two scientists at King's College London, Rosalind Franklin and Maurice Wilkins, began to try and capture an image of a DNA molecule to understand its form and structure. In 1953, Franklin took what was considered one of the most perfect images of the wet form of DNA, referred to as Photograph 51. Wilkins showed a young biologist named James Watson this image, and this convinced Watson that DNA was made of two intertwined helical structures. He and his colleague Francis Crick went on to create the perfect model and publish a paper which changed biology forever, heralding the birth of the new science of genetics. This chapter came to its conclusion with the complete mapping of the entire human genome by the late 1990s, which required global collaboration among hundreds of scientists and cost billions of dollars. But finally, the book of life was wide open, offering us its pages to read and even tinker with.

Progress has continued unabated and we now have a much deeper understanding of different genes and of how they affect traits and diseases. Scientists routinely sequence the mutated genes of cancer patients for more precisely targeted medication. They have achieved a major breakthrough with a new gene editing tool called CRISPR, which allows us to edit a gene down to a single letter. And just to put this into perspective: we're talking about the equivalent of a single word in a genetic code that is spelled by three billion letters. In fact, over half of the nearly 30,000 diseases that are caused due to genetic malfunctions are caused by a single letter in a single gene being out of place. Imagine how marvellous it would be to surgically fix the damaged letter and kill the disease for good!

It is now possible to do a basic genetic test for a few thousand rupees, and to get your entire genome sequenced for less than fifty thousand rupees. You can learn about your genetic disposition, how your genes affect your health and how you can counter these effects with lifestyle changes. If you are the curious type, you can even trace your genetic lineage all the way to the Neanderthals—to understand what percentage of your genes comes from this sister species of the *Homo sapiens* that went extinct 30,000 years ago, but not before interbreeding with our own species, and leaving their signatures in our genetic fingerprints.

The field of genetics can help promote healthier lifestyles and prevent disease, and is becoming more mainstream. With a deep and personalized knowledge of how our genes affect our health, a brand-new chapter in the story of health is slowly but surely beginning.

5. Influential Health Studies

Despite the overwhelming number of health fads and trends that come and go, there are also, fortunately, many serious scientists who have been studying health and lifestyle through rigorous, double-blind, placebo-controlled and often long-term studies. A few of these have become significant landmarks, making big contributions to what we now know about good health.

The China Study

In the 1980s, an expansive study of nutrition, lifestyle and disease was undertaken with 6,500 adult subjects from 130 villages across rural China, jointly funded by Cornell University, the University of Oxford and the Chinese Academy of Preventive Medicine. This turned out to be one of the most comprehensive research studies of all time on the connections between diet, health and disease.[8] At the time, the common belief was that malnutrition in children was caused by a lack of access to protein, particularly 'high quality animal protein'. However, in one of its most significant findings, the study discovered that childhood growth rates in the study regions had significantly increased in the decades preceding 1980, despite the fact that most subjects' diets had only 3–6 per cent of total calories coming from protein. It also found that increased body size was related to higher intake of plant protein, and not animal protein, as is the common assumption.

In his book *The China Study*, T. Colin Campbell, one of the study's lead researchers, makes a case for a plant-based diet, providing evidence for the relationship between animal protein and disease, including cancer. In the study, he found that the Chinese people who ate the most animal protein had a higher incidence of what he called 'diseases of affluence' or 'Western diseases', such as cancer, diabetes and coronary artery disease.

Modern science has confirmed that plant-based diets, in which we get a majority of our calories from plant sources, have numerous health benefits, but animal protein, especially when organic, antibiotic-free, grass-fed and free-range, has its own place in our diets for those who want it.

Framingham Study

In the 1940s, cardiovascular disease had become America's number one killer, and yet the medical establishment lacked a proper understanding of the disease. After Franklin D. Roosevelt's death in 1945 from heart disease that had gone undiagnosed for years, President Harry Truman introduced the National Heart Act, which established the National Heart Institute and set up a grant for a long-term epidemiological heart study. The town of Framingham in Massachusetts was chosen as the site for the study.[9]

The first cohort of 5,209 men and women between the ages of thirty and sixty-two were recruited in 1948, and the first major findings were published in 1957, highlighting the role played by hypertension in coronary heart disease and stroke.

The Framingham Study resulted in a shift in our approach to heart disease, from treatment to prevention. Some of the key findings of the study included:

- High cholesterol levels increased likelihood of heart disease
- Cigarette smoking increased risk of heart disease
- High levels of HDL cholesterol—the good cholesterol—reduced the risk of death
- Enlarged left ventricle correlated to increased risk of stroke
- Obesity is a risk factor in heart disease
- Diabetes is associated with higher risk for heart disease and heart failure

Seventy years later, the study continues, as one of the longest running epidemiological surveys.

The Seven Countries Study

In 1958, physiologist Ancel Keys conceived and implemented a longitudinal epidemiological study called the Seven Countries Study to study the relationships between diet, lifestyle and heart disease. To gauge if cultural differences in nutrition and lifestyle affected heart disease and stroke, seven countries were chosen for this study: the USA, the Netherlands, Italy, Greece, Finland, former Yugoslavia and Japan. The study chose 12,763 men aged between forty and fifty-nine. Among several other results, the study showed that serum cholesterol, blood pressure, diabetes and smoking are risk factors in coronary artery disease.

One of the better-known outcomes of the Seven Countries Study was the popularity of the Mediterranean Diet. The fact that Greece and Italy had better heart health than other regions in the study led Keys and his team to believe that the secret lay in their diet that was rich in vegetables, grain, nuts, seeds, whole foods and olive oil. While the study has faced criticism and controversy, it remains the first of its kind that pointed to the fact that heart health is related to lifestyle, environment and diet.[10]

The Nurses' Health Study

The Nurses' Health Study, which began in 1976 and is now in its third generation of subjects, is one of the largest investigations into chronic disease in women. It was established by Dr Frank Speizer, with the initial objective of studying the long-term effects of oral contraceptives and smoking on breast cancer. In the years and cohorts that followed, the scope of the study expanded to include thirty chronic diseases.

The Nurses Health Studies have had a profound impact on health and healthcare, tracing the effects of cigarette smoking, oral contraceptives, obesity, alcohol, diet and physical activity on breast cancer, coronary heart disease, stroke, hip fracture and eye function, among others. Some of the key findings of the NHS have been:

- Cigarette smoking increases risk of colon cancer and hip fracture
- Obesity increases the risk for heart disease, breast cancer, colon cancer and cataract
- Moderate consumption of alcohol reduces risk of heart disease and cognitive impairment; increased consumption increases risks for cancer
- High consumption of red meat increases the risk of premenopausal breast cancer and colon cancer
- A diet high in vegetables, especially green, leafy vegetables, reduces the risk of cognitive impairment
- Physical activity reduces risk of breast cancer, colon cancer, heart disease, hip fracture and cognitive impairment

The Apple Heart Study

Health studies are also keeping up with the times. In November 2017, Apple and Stanford Medicine launched the Apple Heart Study, using data from Apple Watch to see if wearable devices could track irregularities in heart rhythm, particularly atrial fibrillation. The virtual study had more than 4,00,000 participants, and preliminary results showed that the Apple Watch technology could safely identify irregularities.[11] This truly opens up a whole world of innovation, in which wearable devices aren't just trackers, but also play a potential role in prevention and prediction. In September 2019, Apple announced plans to launch three more health studies in which participants will be users of the Apple Watch who want to contribute to the research.[12] The studies are the Apple Women's Health Study, the Apple Hearing Study and the Apple Heart and Movement Study. The coming together of technology and health is a symbol of the future of global healthcare.

We are lucky to live at a time when science is working hard to decipher how health works, translating findings into simple choices for us. What is also incredible is that these findings often validate conventional wisdom that people have been following for centuries, such as hiking up a mountain for a pilgrimage, observing periods of silence or practicing fasting rituals.

6. Discovering Our Defences

In Greek mythology, disease descended upon the world when Pandora opened the box given to her as a wedding present by Zeus, unable to heed his warning never to open it. Along with greed, pain, hunger, poverty, war and death, illness was unleashed onto the world of humans. For much of human history, disease was thought to be caused by evil spirits, or as punishment for immoral behaviour and sin. Hippocrates, the Greek physician was one of the first to go beyond superstition, explaining illness as a result of an imbalance between the four humours that he identified in the body.

Between the fourteenth and eighteenth centuries, as epidemics began to rage through populations, two theories arose to explain the spread of illness through a community. The first attributed disease to miasma, or 'bad air', poisonous vapours emitting from rotting organic material. The second theory was known as contagion, which was based on the observation that diseases like smallpox spread from person to person. It was an English physician, John Snow, who found that cholera in nineteenth century London was actually spread through contaminated water. This paved the way for the emergence of the germ theory of illness, a revolutionary idea that still underlies our study of immunity today. Robert Koch, at the end of the nineteenth century, proved that germs could cause disease, by injecting anthrax bacteria taken from the blood of a cow that had died from the disease into a mouse, which then contracted the illness.

Various fascinating discoveries and studies have helped advance our understanding of immunity to the point we're at today, but the concept of the vaccine was one of the major turning points. In 1721, the British royal family was anxious—in the way perhaps royals often were—about the smallpox epidemic affecting their own children. At the time, it was known that someone once infected with the smallpox virus wouldn't contract the illness again, and so a 'clinical trial' was carried out. Six convicts, faced with the choice of participating or being executed, 'volunteered' to have skin and pus from a smallpox patient rubbed into incisions on their arms and legs. All developed mild symptoms for a few days and then recovered. The trial, however questionable it was ethically, was considered a success, and the Prince and Princess of Wales had two of their daughters inoculated against the virus. In other similar instances of inoculation, however, a small percentage of people died. Fast-forward to 1796, when Edward Jenner observed that milkmaids never contracted smallpox and assumed this was because of their exposure to the much less virulent cowpox virus. He extracted pus from a dairymaid who had been infected with cowpox, and inoculated his gardener's eight-year-old son. When the little boy was given pus from a smallpox patient, he didn't fall ill. This moment is believed to mark the birth of immunology. The term 'vaccine' was coined by the surgeon Richard Dunning, from the Latin word *vacca* meaning 'cow'. The march of progress continued and eventually smallpox was eradicated for good in 1989.

History is filled with happy accidents that helped us understand our body's defences, but what is ultimately clear is that our immune system is truly an elegantly designed one, one that might just need us to cooperate better in the modern world.

HEALTH HACK #4: Haldi for Health

Growing up in India, we've all been fed turmeric in various forms—in warm milk, in hot water with honey and in every meal. Recently, the West has gotten in on the secret thanks to modern research validating ancient wisdom. Curcumin, the main compound in turmeric, has anti-inflammatory and anti-ageing properties, boosting heart and brain health. Remember, though, that for the body to absorb all its goodness, turmeric needs to be consumed along with pepper and a source of fat.

---

7. THE RISE OF EXERCISE

Movement was intrinsic to human life for most of our history, but the idea of consciously exercising for better health might date back to 2500 B.C. China. The teachings of Confucius mentioned the need to engage in physical activity to avoid 'stoppages' or 'organ malfunction'. This eventually led to the development of 'Cong Fu' gymnastics, likely taught by Taoist priests, which involved different movements, postures and breathing to keep the body functioning optimally.[13] In India, Yoga is believed to have originated at least 5,000 years ago.

Through history, levels of physical fitness rose and fell, ebbing and flowing with ancient civilizations. In many empires, exercise was central to having able and battle-ready armies, so young boys and men would join rigorous training programmes involving horse riding, hunting, marching and other activities. As individual empires—from Persia to Rome—grew wealthier and more stable, however, there was often a drop in fitness levels, as populations turned from military and physical matters to matters of the court, indulging in corruption, entertainment and material excesses.

Ancient Greece had a unique relationship with physical fitness. Based on the idea of 'a sound mind in a sound body', and an appreciation for the beauty of the human form, there was a great deal of focus on achieving levels of physical perfection through exercise. The Father of Modern Medicine, Hippocrates, and other ancient Greek physicians also prescribed movement for health reasons. Young boys joined organized facilities for physical education, with a focus on running, jumping and wrestling. Sparta was known for creating the perfect warriors, with intensive training programmes for boys right from the age of six. While women were rarely included in the rigours of physical training in Sparta, their health and physical fitness were important from the perspective of producing strong children who would join the state.

The tradition of strongmen in Europe foreshadowed the dawn of body building in the early twentieth century, which saw a shift in focus from acts of strength like lifting a horse off the ground, to the aesthetics of a muscular body. With the explosive rise of

Arnold Schwarzenegger and the iconic Gold's Gym on Venice Beach in California, bodybuilding changed the way we looked at the human body. Other revolutionary trendsetters in global fitness include the likes of Jack LaLanne and Jane Fonda, whose fitness videos on television were far ahead of their times. Fonda inspired an entire generation of women to exercise in the privacy of their homes. Unfortunately, fitness for women has always been closely tied to specific body shapes and weights which has caused eating disorders and unrealistic beauty standards that our society has still not entirely overcome.

Despite the rise of new kinds of workouts, for many people up until the end of the turn of the millennium, health and fitness was synonymous with hitting the gym and lifting weights. But there was a fatal flaw in this. The modern gym as it was, was designed for bodybuilding, an aesthetic sport. Doing bench presses or bicep curls has very little to do with long-term health and thankfully, we know better now and a modern health aficionado has a much broader variety of solutions to pick from.

HEALTH HACK #5: Infrared and Red Light Therapy

Red and infrared light have been found to be effective tools for muscle recovery and pain relief, with the potential to treat inflammation and play a role in detoxification and treatment for other kinds of illness and injury. This cutting-edge technology is now available in the form of compact lamps for home use.

8. DIET FADS

If the gym was the most visible sign of the rising interest in health, the fad diet was its evil twin. You would start one 'amazing' diet, just about getting the hang of it before it morphed into something different, growing ever more elusive, and ultimately taking you right back to what you had been doing all along.

The allure of a magic diet that delivers on numerous health goals in a few weeks is hard to resist, and I speak from experience, having tried almost every diet over the last twenty years, and experienced innumerable failures to show for it.

One of the first blockbuster diets was the Atkins diet, named after Dr Robert Atkins whose book *The New Diet Revolution* sold over fifteen million copies. Atkins advocated severe carb restrictions, with users deriving most calories from fats and proteins. Followers often gleefully have multiple servings of bacon and steak, and still lose weight in the short run. But strictly following this diet causes many long-term health issues and most people eventually give up on it.[14]

The GM diet which has found popular appeal is a kind of crash diet that can lead to a loss of 3–5 kg in a week or two. The diet recommends vegetables and fruits in specific configurations while restricting calories to very few sources. The resulting shock indeed leads to weight loss, but the diet is seldom sustainable and is highly unbalanced in the long run.[15]

There have been many variations of paleo diets, supposedly mimicking the diets of our hunter–gatherer ancestors. They focus on eating raw, seasonal fruits and vegetables and naturally raised animal protein. The paleo diet definitely gets the fundamentals right and might be worth drawing from, to construct the ideal diet for your health goals.

The keto diet, the latest craze, is similar to Atkins but focuses more on healthy fats. It is based on a more scientific approach to get the body into ketosis, a state in which ketones are used as alternatives to glucose as the primary fuel source.

While most of these diets are not sustainable or effective beyond the short-term, the upside is the increased awareness about nutrition—with every new fad, a new horde of followers is recruited, who end up developing awareness and insights about what and how they should and shouldn't eat.

HEALTH HACK #6: Skip a Meal

If you find diets impossibly hard to sustain, just skip a meal. If you're nervous about skipping a meal, start by going a few hours longer without food in between meals, or having a really light dinner like a bowl of soup or dal. Eventually you can start skipping breakfast or dinner altogether, and even do twenty-four-hour fasts once or twice a week.

---

9. GREEK GOD CELEBRITIES

We live in the age of the influencer. It is estimated that 4.15 billion people use social media worldwide[16] and the number is rising rapidly. It isn't a surprise then, that social media 'influencers' wield an incredible amount of influence over almost every aspect of our lives. And health is no exception. Instagram is filled with fitness celebrities with chiselled six packs and beach bodies that millions of people follow every day and aspire to emulate.

At the same time, our movie stars and sports heroes are getting fitter than ever. In fact, the most talked about aspect of a film is often how hard an actor worked to achieve a particular body—athletic or super chiselled—to fit a character. Think about Farhan Akhtar's look in *Bhaag Milkha Bhaag* or Priyanka Chopra's transformation for the film *Mary Kom*. These movies inspire millions of fans to pursue similar levels of fitness.

In India, one of the most memorable of these transformations is that of Virat Kohli, the captain of the Indian cricket team. Cricketers had never really been known for their fitness, but after the 2012 IPL, Kohli realized that, to be on top of his game, he really needed to change his life around. Over the next few years, he lost 11 or 12 kg, by completely overhauling his habits. He changed his diet, began to spend many hours training in the gym everyday and focused on getting better sleep. This visible change that fans observed in one of India's cricket greats sparked a new interest in fitness and healthy lifestyles.

Many Bollywood fans might remember Kareena Kapoor's size zero phase, where she lost 8 kg for the film *Tashan*. She did this with the help of experts for a specific role, but the 'size zero' fad became an unhealthy obsession for many, especially young women. While celebrities and influencers have undoubtedly begun to promote the culture of fitness, there is potential for fans to fixate on unrealistic aesthetic goals. It's important for people in positions of influence to emphasize the idea of holistic wellness rather than short-term or superficial goals, by highlighting the importance of sleep, working out and good nutrition. Fortunately, there are also celebrity influencers on social media who are promoting a more body-positive culture, embracing bodies of all shapes and sizes.

10. Lifestyle Diseases

In the early twentieth century, a missionary doctor named Samuel Hutton was working in Nain on the northern coast of Labrador in Canada. He observed that the locals in the region could be divided into two groups—one consisting of people who lived isolated from European populations and ate a traditional diet, and the other who lived in Nain or closer to European settlements and had started consuming what he called a 'settler's diet', of tea, bread, biscuits, molasses, salt fish and pork. In the first group, Hutton had never seen or heard of a case of cancer, asthma, or other 'Western' diseases, while those in the latter, he noticed, came to him with complaints of scurvy, weakness and fatigue far more often.[17] This might have been one of the earliest observations of something we have become all too familiar with—lifestyle diseases, also called non-communicable diseases (NCDs) since they are caused by lifestyle factors.

While modern medicine has ensured that we no longer die of infections and lifespans have nearly doubled in the last 150 years, lifestyle diseases have significantly cut down what is known as health span, or the number of disease-free years one has. We have begun to think of lifestyle diseases as inevitable, especially after the age of fifty. What we will discover, however, is that we are not helpless in the face of these diseases, and that choosing a healthier lifestyle can prevent, delay and even reverse their symptoms. It is possible to thrive even in older age, living a life of energy, vitality and joy.

11. A Brief History of Mental Health

There was a time when mental illnesses were believed to be caused by demonic possession, or due to the displeasure of the gods. Skulls and cave art from around 6500 BC show evidence of trephination—the drilling of holes in the skull to free evil spirits trapped within that caused mental illness. Rather than doctors, priests were called upon for the treatment of mental illnesses, in the belief that patients needed to repent for their sins and have their demons exorcized. In ancient Egypt and Mesopotamia, it was believed that, in women, a wandering uterus pressing against various organs around the body led to mental illness. The recommended treatment method to lure the uterus back into position was the use of substances with pleasant smells and sneezing.[18] The perceptions surrounding mental health were thus steeped in the supernatural and tied closely to morality and shame. Rather than seen as being unwell, people with mental illnesses were thought to have committed sins or wronged the gods.

It was only in 400 B.C. that Hippocrates began to separate the world of superstition and religion from the health of the body and mind. He put forward the theory that all illnesses stemmed from either a deficiency or excess in one of four bodily fluids, called the humours—blood, yellow bile, black bile and phlegm. Hippocrates was also one of the first to classify types of mental illness as epilepsy, mania, melancholy and brain fever. Despite the field undergoing positive changes thanks to the work of the great Greek physicians, those living with mental illnesses continued to suffer through the ages. For example, in order to balance the humours, doctors often practiced bloodletting on their patients, using leeches. In medieval Europe, natural disasters and outbreaks of diseases were blamed on the supernatural, and often women with some form of mental illness were cast as the villains, resulting in terrible witch hunts and killings. In the fifteenth century, with the establishment of asylums and institutions, the so-called 'insane' were incarcerated with criminals and other 'undesirable' elements of society, and treated in an inhumane manner: a reflection of how the world saw them. In overcrowded and unhygienic institutions, patients were often 'treated' with isolation, restraint and occasionally even more brutal methods that involved forms of physical violence.

Finally, the nineteenth century saw the rise of psychology as a field of study and practice, with various forms of therapy being used to treat mental illnesses. Even though we now have cutting-edge science to help us better understand and address mental health, stigma continues to remain attached to many aspects of this field of health.

12. BIOHACKING

What if we were to view the human body as a system, like other systems, whose parameters we can tinker with to change how we feel, perform and age? Add a supplement here, track your sleep there, and maybe even undergo some cryotherapy—and voila, you are officially biohacking. DIY biology is currently all the rage, especially in places like Silicon Valley and Hollywood. The term encompasses everything from taking supplements, tracking sleep, exercise and nutrition in minute detail, to some pretty extreme activities like using cryotherapy or ozone therapy. Biohackers are those who experiment on themselves to find ways to drastically boost their physical and cognitive performance, and to live longer. Much of this experimentation happens outside of institutional settings, and involves citizen scientists spending time and money on research and trials. The field is controversial because many of the treatments used are not officially recognized by medical institutions or governing bodies.

I recently had the good fortune of meeting Ben Greenfield, one of the most influential biohackers of our time. His latest book

Boundless: Upgrade Your Brain, Optimize Your Body & Defy Ageing is an excellent guided tour for everything cutting-edge in the field of biohacking. Ben's book has outstanding insights into boosting performance and health by leveraging the latest from science and offering practical tips for a beginner biohacker.

Another well-known biohacker who is really pushing the envelope is Dave Asprey. Asprey is quite convinced that with the right lifestyle, supplements, medication and other means of hacking his biology, he could live to the age of 180. And towards that end, he has turned himself into a guinea pig for his own experiments. Among other things, Asprey has spent thousands of dollars ordering pig whipworm eggs (a parasite that cannot reproduce in humans) in order to reduce inflammation in the gut and improve immunity and has also undergone stem cell therapy (a procedure he livestreamed on Facebook!) which helped him heal from old injuries.

Biohackers are like the pioneers of old, who set out to find new lands and adventures, often at great peril to their own lives and wellbeing. They are willing to take calculated risks, try new things on themselves and share their findings with larger audiences. Although biohacking is certainly pushing the boundaries of what we know about health, and some of the practices from this subculture will eventually find their way into the mainstream, a lot of the findings have not yet gone through the gold standard of placebo-controlled, double-blind studies. For this reason, it could be a long time before we understand the risks and benefits more precisely.

But for the adventurous among us, this is certainly an exciting area and there is a lot to try if you do your homework well, use only the best brands and clinics and consult with your doctor. I am certainly open to trying out new supplements, immunity-boosting therapies, miracle compounds often derived from ancient herbs and new recovery therapies.

13. Chasing Immortality

The idea of immortality is one that has fascinated humanity since the beginning of time. We all dream of overcoming the decrepitude of old age, even of escaping death to live forever. The gods and heroes of our legends who live eternally reflect this deep desire; the stories of their lives told in eons that are unfathomable to us with our ordinary human lifespans. Immortality has always had a magical quality, inspiring awe and flights of fancy. Humans of every age have dreamt of discovering the elixir of eternal youth or a magic potion that can defeat death itself. Some have even tried earnestly to make these dreams a reality, guided by vague references in ancient texts, revelations that came to them in dreams, or by myths that they took all too seriously.

One of the oldest pieces of literature in the world, the Mesopotamian Epic of Gilgamesh, also features a quest for immortality. Gilgamesh, the King of Uruk, abandons his kingdom and sets out on his epic journey after the death of his best friend Enkidu. After many adventures and challenges, he ultimately fails in his search for eternal life, but he has a profound epiphany when he realizes that while he might not live forever, humankind will.

It seems we are consumed by the idea of breaking the bonds of our mortality and living forever. So, on the one hand, our myths and legends illustrate this in beautiful poetry and prose that will last forever.

On the other hand, we have been making steady progress in the field of medicine, conquering one disease after another, dramatically extending human lifespan and cracking the code of genes, the language that life is written in. People have started to think beyond what seems currently plausible and are now seriously asking what truly is the limit of the human lifespan. We don't know that answer yet, but there have been many tantalizing experiments with animals in labs that have prolonged life considerably, enough to catch the attention of mainstream scientists and entrepreneurs.

For me personally, a big Aha! moment came when I read Ray Kurzweil's book *Fantastic Voyage: Live Long Enough to Live Forever*. One might be forgiven for thinking of Kurzweil as a bit of an eccentric, if it were not for the fact that he is also an inventor of impeccable repute, the founder of Singularity University and Director of Engineering at Google. With the pace at which we are making progress with engineering our underlying biology, Kurzweil believes that it won't be long before we can transcend biology and dramatically increase the human lifespan.

Many scientists and entrepreneurs have taken Ray's vision seriously enough to invest billions of dollars in cutting-edge research and companies, with the stated goal of curing ageing or even eventually solving death. Google's founders have invested in Calico, a company that wants to harness technology to understand and increase human lifespan. The company Human Longevity is working on understanding the genetic underpinning of ageing to find therapies that slow it down. Recently, Elizabeth Blackburn won a Nobel Prize for her research into how shortened telomeres, protective caps at the end of our DNA, play a significant role in ageing. Her company, Teloyears, even sells a testing kit to measure the length of your telomeres, as well as supplements to slow down their deterioration.

David Sinclair is professor of Genetics in Harvard University and best known for his research on the anti-ageing effects of resveratrol. In his recent bestselling book *Lifespan*, he explains the cutting-edge science of ageing and how certain chemicals like NMN and metformin can have significant benefits as anti-ageing drugs. Sinclair, however, emphasizes the idea of prolonging vitality rather than simply extending life. It is not merely about living more years, but about remaining healthy and thriving through those years.

This brings us to the end of our quick tour of the story of health. From the benign beginnings of measuring a lowly calorie to the world of fad diets, from dealing with lifestyle diseases to chasing immortality, from Greek god physiques to increasing health spans, from paleo lifestyles to genetics, this story has come a long way. We know more about health than any generation before us. Armed with the knowledge of this evolving story, we can appreciate how the modern narrative came to be and we can pursue health in a deliberate and systematic manner without succumbing to the lure of quick fixes. Now that we have a big picture understanding, let's dive into all the building blocks for good health and see how we can craft a game plan suitable to each of our individual aspirations.

In Summary

1. Once used by the US government to ration food and by popular health experts to promote weight loss, the lowly calorie has had a fascinating history.

2. Beware the hidden interests of food lobbies that try to sell us foods high in unhealthy sugars and empty calories in the guise of low-fat and healthy products.

3. Sleep science transformed how we perceive night-time rest, with the discovery of the circadian rhythm and impact of sleep phases on memory, learning and overall health.

4. The story of the discovery of the gene is the stuff of legend, and rapid progress in recent decades has shown us its profound role in the future of health.

5. Long-term health studies over the last century have revolutionized our understanding of health and lifestyle diseases, continuing to inform diagnosis and treatment.

6. Early theories of immunity ranged from the mythical to the abstract, but drawing from epidemics and the spread of infections, more robust science emerged.

7. Organized forms of exercise rose and fell with empires, while the tradition of strongmen led to the bodybuilding movement, and then to the modern gym as we now know it.

8. From Atkins and GM to paleo and keto, diets have long been sold as miracle weight loss solutions, and yet, most are not sustainable or effective in the long run.

9. While influencers and celebrities can help draw attention to good health through their platforms, they also promote unrealistic goals and unhealthy obsessions with weight.

10. Virtually non-existent in communities following traditional ways of life, lifestyle diseases seem to go hand-in-hand with a Western lifestyle and diet.

11. For centuries, mental health was misunderstood and mired in superstition, resulting in torturous treatment methods and witch hunts, until the rise of psychology in the 1800s.

12. Biohackers operate on the fringe, experimenting with supplements, technologies and treatments to measure and hack their bodies for better health.

13. Immortality has been a long-cherished dream, evidenced in many myths and legends, and research now tells us that longer and healthier lives might just be within our reach.

PART 2
THE BASICS

3

FOOD & DIETS

There is no food neutral; there is no food Switzerland—every single thing you put in your mouth is either making you more healthy or less healthy.—Dallas and Melissa Hartwig, *It Starts with Food*

Let food be thy medicine and medicine be thy food.—Hippocrates

There was a time in my life when I was going to the gym regularly, focusing on building muscle and buffing up, as they say. In addition to lifting weights at the gym as often as I could, I was also taking several supplements and increasing my protein intake. The advice back then for people wanting to bulk up was to eat six times a day, and make sure all of those meals had some form of protein. So that's what I did. In fact, I followed the advice so closely that I also made sure to have casein—a slow digesting protein—just before I went to sleep at night. The idea behind this way of eating was to provide the body with the nutrition it needed right through a twenty-four-hour cycle, in order to repair and build muscle.

Fast forward to today, and the science of nutrition has drastically changed. In fact, study after scientific study has now proved how little food we need for good health, and how important it is to have long windows of not eating in every twenty-four-hour cycle. Intermittent fasting—going 14–16 hours without food everyday—is now known to streamline the body's glucose mechanism to keep blood sugar in check and to train the body's fat metabolism to function better.

For some years, I had been reading about the science of fasting, and I grew convinced that this was something I needed to incorporate into my lifestyle for better health. However, every time I tried to fast, I struggled. Even skipping breakfast was hard and felt nearly impossible. In my mind, breakfast was the most important meal of the day. And so, every year, I would try to increase my fasting periods, only to give up.

As time went by and I read more of the research on the science of intermittent fasting, I decided I needed to push myself harder. I told myself I'd gradually increase my fasting windows and try to sustain this for at least a week. After just one week of intermittent fasting, however, I felt low on energy. I struggled with my workouts and felt tired all the time. By this point of time, I was almost ready to accept that intermittent fasting was just not for me. Instead of experiencing the much advertised bursts of high energy, I had to contend with persistent fatigue, leading to bouncing back to even deeper carb binges—and so it went for a while.

Fortunately, before I gave up completely, I came across more literature on the subject, from which I learnt two important things. The first was that one needs to sustain an intermittent fasting plan for at least three to four weeks for the body to get used to it.

Basically, I hadn't given my body a chance to adapt to this new eating plan. Secondly, I learnt that there are several non-caloric drinks one can consume during the fasting window, which helped me get through the longer hours of not eating. I concocted various lemon-based drinks to get me through the periods of craving until the next eating window. I gradually increased the fasting window by just one hour every few days, until I was able to increase it to sixteen hours. I recently even did a twenty-four-hour fast— something unthinkable for me even a short while ago—and felt pretty good while doing it! Two meals a day has become standard for me, and I might even skip one of those if I feel like it. The realization that food at times is optional and your body can rely on both internal and external sources for calories has been absolutely liberating! This is not to say I don't enjoy a cheat meal of masala dosa in the morning every now and then! After all, Bangalore is famous for buzzing breakfast places like MTR, whose dosas are to die for!

The biggest lesson from my fasting journey has been patience— not only giving the body time to adjust to the way it's being fed, but also time for the mind, which is so conditioned to think that three meals a day are critical for our survival, to adapt. It is through this trial and error over a long period of time and also devouring (no calories here!) copious amounts of literature on this subject, that I now have a better understanding of the scientifically complex but intuitively simple practice of healthy eating. Let's dive in.

* * *

Every discussion of a healthy lifestyle begins and ends with food. Food is the vital force that drives life, a source of energy that fuels our bodies, and yet it is also so much more. It is an integral part of our social fabric, bringing families and loved ones together, marking special occasions and evoking memory and nostalgia. It is also powerfully linked to identity. For a moment, just think of a freshly fried kachori, a fluffy naan or a plate of exquisite, handmade sushi—it is likely that each conjures an entire story, of culture, flavour, geography and identity.

Food nourishes our bodies and our brains. In fact, food might have shaped our evolution as human beings. The moment our ancestors began to cook food, thanks to the discovery of fire, was the moment that changed the course of our history. There is now a school of thought that believes that the shift to a diet of cooked foods coincided with the increase in the size of the human brain. Cooking allowed us to extract more calories than we could from raw sources of food, fuelling the energy-guzzling organ that was our growing brain. The changes in the way our ancestors ate might have also altered our social behaviour—from gender roles to family units. Food truly is integral to the human experience.

There is a fleeting moment in *Man's Search for Meaning*, Viktor Frankl's memoir of his time in Nazi concentration camps, that is at once poignant and telling about our relationship with food. Frankl remembers how, whenever prisoners found themselves working without a guard hovering over them, their talk would turn to food. They were terribly undernourished, yet driven by memories and thoughts of food, animatedly discussing their favourite dishes and what they would cook for each other at a reunion in the future. As heart-wrenching as this image is—of starving prisoners torn from their lives and loved ones, being subjected daily to humiliation, dreaming of food even as their bodies were wasting away—it is also a powerful reminder that hunger is both a primitive desire for survival and a link to emotions of comfort and familiarity. Perhaps it is useful to remind ourselves once in a while—as we shop for groceries, as we cook a meal for a loved one, or as we laugh with friends over a delicious meal—that food is nourishment in more ways than one.

Over the years, our relationship with food has become complicated, and the modern obsession with fads and diets doesn't make things any easier. It's almost funny, when you think about the fact that eating, which is something every single organism has been doing intuitively and effortlessly for billions of years, has suddenly become a source of controversy and stress for us, the highly educated and advanced inhabitants of the twenty-first century. So complex has our approach to food become, that it seems we just cannot make up our minds about what to eat!

In some ways, our approach to food has come full circle over the last several decades. We went from eating what our grandparents traditionally ate, to eating what the modern Western world was eating and gradually are now relearning what our ancestors knew. We went from eating ghee with every meal to villainizing all fats to suddenly rediscovering how healthful certain fats like ghee and coconut oil are for us. Ghee has even started to do the rounds as the new superfood, and rightly so, as we now know that saturated fats are an integral part of healthy and balanced diets. The rise of Bulletproof coffee has even made the habit of pouring butter or coconut oil into your morning coffee, uber-cool!

Michael Pollan, who has written some of the finest books on food, asserts that food science, or what he calls 'nutritionism', has alienated us so completely from food itself, that we need to relearn some of the basics when it comes to what we eat. His advice: 'Eat food. Not too much. Mostly plants.'[1] He also advises not to eat anything your grandmother wouldn't, to avoid buying products with more than five ingredients and to avoid food products that make a health claim, as it is likely to be based on questionable science. It is for a good reason that most of us in India love our home food, even though we may overdo it around festivals!

Reducing the rich histories and experiences of food and eating to its nutritional parts—fats, carbs, proteins, vitamins and more—helped us forget how to feed ourselves. And so, nutritionists, food scientists, food lobbies, dieticians and books began to replace the wisdom of our mothers and grandmothers, who had learnt to cook with fresh, seasonal, local ingredients that balanced each other perfectly in traditional recipes. I remember being able to eat bhindi for only short summer months and sarson-ka-saag only in winter months, as per the seasonal availability. Suddenly, we had to seek the advice of experts for something that our species had been doing instinctively, and pretty well, if you ask me, for its entire existence.

As I continue to experiment with my nutrition, I have come to realize that food is about so much more than physical nourishment or providing the body with energy in the form of calories. Food also has a huge psychological element. It is intrinsically tied to our state of mind, our moods and emotions. There are days I just want to eat something familiar—comfort foods that immediately make me feel better, often going against all the nutrition advice I have read and heard. I truly believe that different things work for different people. While being disciplined about a healthy lifestyle is important, rigidity is rarely sustainable. What works best for me is following some basic ground rules when it comes to eating, while remaining flexible and adapting to different situations.

As we get down to some of the more practical details of diet and nutrition, while learning how to make better food choices, we will try not to lose sight of the fact that eating healthy, tasty and nutritious meals can and should be a pleasurable experience.

What's Wrong with the Modern Diet

*The most important thing to remember about food labels is that
you should avoid foods that have labels.*—Joel Fuhrman

In the modern world, certain things have taken priority over
others when it comes to shopping for, cooking and eating food.
At the top of this list are convenience and speed. Living in nuclear
families, working long hours and battling packed schedules, most
of us want to find shortcuts when it comes to preparing meals for
ourselves and our families. Enter the pre-packaged drive-through
fast food meal and even the ready-to-eat upma or rajma chawal
that just requires adding boiling water to a cup! Of course, these
meals are usually inexpensive and save us huge amounts of time (let
alone effort and washing up), but what have we lost in the process?
Perhaps asking this question can help us answer another—what is
wrong with our modern diets?

Before getting into nutritional specifics, it's important to
pause and think of what food means to us beyond nutrition. Food
has always been an integral part of identity and culture. Culinary
traditions are unique to every region and have been passed down
through generations. Learning how to cook used to involve
understanding seasonal ingredients, local produce and varied
flavours, and balancing the health effects of each ingredient. Food
ties families together, defines communities and is a great source
of comfort. Think about your favourite meal that your parents
or grandparents cooked for you, perhaps on a birthday or a
special occasion. You'll probably be flooded with memories—the
fragrances of spices wafting out of the kitchen, the delicious flavours
and the laughter that accompanied them at the dining table. This
is what food can be—a rich, social and deeply fulfilling experience.

Now fast-forward to the meal you most often eat in the middle of a workday or on a weekend. Do you usually grab a sandwich to eat at your desk for lunch? Perhaps you pick up a roll or make some instant noodles for dinner and order in biriyani when there's a birthday in the family. There's absolutely no judgement if you do any of these; you aren't to blame for choosing convenience over everything else. We live in a time of high stress and busy schedules. Add to that the industrialization of the food industry and the easy access to a vast array of instant foods, sugary drinks and snacks, and the story unfolds completely. Pause and think for a second about what's the most frequently ordered dish on Swiggy and Zomato! Who would have thought that biryani will top all charts all over the country as the most frequent indulgence!

Given that many of us, living in urban areas, seem to have lost the deep connections with food that were forged growing up or that faded away in our parents' generation, we're all too familiar with the modern diet, also called the Western diet. The Western diet is characterized by refined sugars and grains, highly processed or industrialized foods, genetically modified vegetables, antibiotic-injected meat, deep fried snacks, sweetened beverages and a whole lot of things that don't even remotely resemble naturally occurring foods, but have long shelf lives and are accessible and quick to prepare. A lot of these are simply not nutritious and do not fuel a healthy lifestyle. They leave us craving more sugar or fat, while we feel unsatisfied, heavy and low on energy. There is now sufficient evidence that the modern diet has powerful adverse effects on almost every aspect of our bodies, from immunity to heart health. It has led to what's been termed the pandemic of obesity, as well as a sharp rise in lifestyle diseases such as diabetes, cardiovascular disease and more.

Now that it's clear what's wrong with the modern diet, how can we fix this and create a new modern diet that is holistic and healthy in the long term? It's important not just to change the food we eat, but also to change the way we eat it. Try and create simple rituals around food in your home. Perhaps you and your partner, child or friend can start cooking a meal together once a week. Lay the table, play some music and eat mindfully—paying attention to the flavours and textures of the food. You could also try and recreate recipes from your childhood or find your favourite on YouTube, reviving memories and nostalgia as you make your favourite meals. It's important to make eating an enjoyable experience, rather than one that brings feelings of guilt or shame. And hopefully the rest of this chapter will help you with better food choices to redefine the modern diet.

HEALTH HACK #7: Ditch the Sugar

We now know without a doubt that sugar does absolutely nothing good for our health. In fact, it wreaks havoc with our bodies as well as our minds. So, when it comes to sugar, just skip it! If you're finding it hard, start with having your tea and coffee without sugar, and then gradually start restricting how often you eat dessert. Every time you ditch the sugar, you're earning little brownie points for your health.

A CODE FOR A BALANCED DIET

There is a lot of debate about what is a balanced diet and there have been numerous revisions to the ideal food pyramid, but if you can follow these simple guidelines, you will get all the nutrition that you need:

1. Ensure that you get the majority of your calories from plant-based sources like fruits, vegetables, nuts and seeds, legumes and grains. While fruits and vegetables will provide high quality energy and essential micronutrients, nuts and seeds are packed with healthy fats and proteins.

2. As children, we were berated for not eating our green leafy vegetables, and for good reason. Greens, along with other brightly coloured vegetables like beets, carrots and pumpkins, are packed with all kinds of nutrients, digesting slowly to provide energy for a long time after meals.

3. Incorporate healthy fats that come from ghee, coconut oil, various nut and seed oils, as well as vegetable fat sources like avocado and olive oil. Avoid refined and processed fats such as vegetable oils, margarine and light butter spreads, as well as deep-fried foods, since the cooking process results in the generation of trans fats that can be carcinogenic.

4. Instead of relying only on wheat and rice, get your carbohydrates from diverse sources to make your meals multigrain. Rather than buying multigrain atta, whose ingredients you have no control over, choose grains such as jowar, bajra, makkai, buckwheat, brown rice, ragi, amaranth and quinoa, among several other options.

5. Pulses and legumes, including the dals or lentils so common in an Indian kitchen, as well as chickpeas, black-eyed peas and other beans, are nutrient-rich and a great source of both complex carbohydrates and proteins. Boiled or sprouted pulses are a great addition to any diet.

6. Avoid all kinds of processed foods and sugary drinks like the plague. These are just empty calories that offer no benefits. You might have a dessert or a sweetened drink to celebrate an occasion, but they cannot be part of your everyday diet.

7. Black coffee and all kinds of white and green teas are full
    of flavonoids and antioxidants. These also work as appetite
    suppressants and can be great for your mind. Given that they
    are stimulants, though, it might be a good idea to avoid coffee
    and tea after 4 p.m., especially if you have trouble falling
    asleep.

8. Local and seasonal foods should be a big part of your diet.
    Fruits and vegetables are at their nutritious best and full of
    flavour at the peak of season. One of the best ways to identify
    what is in season is to visit your local vendor who does not
    have a freezer or refrigerator, and to pick what seems to be
    available in abundance and inexpensive.

9. Spices are densely packed pockets of essential micronutrients
    and should be liberally used in your food.

10. Fermented food is a great way to improve the health of the gut.
    In India, these have been an integral part of our diet, from curd
    set at home to rice or cooked vegetables soaked overnight in
    water and pickles. Fermented drinks like kefir and kombucha
    are also great choices.

11. Just because you are eating healthy doesn't mean you
    should be eating all the time. In fact, don't be shy about
    skipping a meal every now and then, to give your gut a
    much needed break.

Food Groups

While we don't always want to reduce food to its parts, it is
important to have a basic understanding of what constitutes the
nutrition our body needs—so here is a very quick overview.

Everything that we eat comes from two major sources:
macronutrients and micronutrients. Macronutrients provide

energy and raw material for the body to function and grow. Micronutrients are trace elements that orchestrate the delicate biochemistry of the body, required in tiny quantities but still essential. There are three major macronutrients— carbohydrates, proteins and fats, all necessary for survival. Alcohol can be considered the fourth macronutrient as it is packed with calories as well, but in a health book, the less we talk about alcohol, the better!

A healthy diet has a balanced mix of all three macronutrients. A general rule of thumb is a 40:30:30 ratio of calories from carbohydrates, proteins and fats, although this might change depending on one's health and goals. It is important to keep in mind that this ratio is by calories, not by weight, which is significant because a gram of carbohydrates and proteins have four calories each, while a gram of fat has nine calories. In other words, a gram of fat provides more than twice as many calories as a gram of carb or protein.

As low-carb and no-carb diets have become all the rage, we sometimes forget that all carbohydrates aren't all bad for us—in fact, they're essential, especially when it comes to fuelling the human brain and our muscles. Carbohydrates are either simple, as in sugars, or complex, as in starches and fibre. Simple carbohydrates, like white bread or doughnuts, might give us an immediate boost of energy, but they leave us feeling hungry soon after, and are therefore considered empty calories. Complex carbohydrates, on the other hand, include fruits, vegetables, legumes and whole grains, all higher in fibre content, digesting slowly and leaving us satisfied. One of the challenges we currently face with our modern diets is that the overwhelming majority of calories comes from refined carbohydrates. They are digested quickly, and lead to unhealthy spikes in sugar levels. By choosing high-fibre, complex carbohydrates, we're nourishing our bodies in the right way, so that we get the energy our bodies need and stay full longer.

Known as the building blocks of life, proteins are essential, a fact recognized by everyone from a bodybuilder trying to gain muscle to a concerned parent of growing children. All proteins are composed of building blocks known as amino acids. Our bodies digest them by breaking them down into their units, before they are transported through the bloodstream to do their jobs—which includes everything from growth and repair to providing energy. While most of us associate protein with egg and meat, vegetarians can get their share from dairy products and pulses. Vegans might need to be a bit more conscious about focusing on other plant-based proteins such as nuts and soya, along with legumes and pulses.

Fat, unfortunately, has been the most maligned macronutrient. The fact that it shares its name with the word we use for the extra weight we carry around hasn't helped—even though the source of that extra weight is usually carbohydrates and sugars, and not fat! Talk about paying for someone else's crimes! Fortunately, in the last decade, fats have been vindicated and even saturated fats have made a full recovery. We now know that fats play a very important role in metabolism and are excellent sources of dense, slow digesting calories. If a nutritious diet is your aim, you must make sure there are enough calories coming from healthy fats. We will take a closer look at how to make fats work to our advantage later in this chapter.

CALORIE BUSINESS

We got acquainted with calories as we took a whirlwind tour of the story of health, and now I want to dig a little deeper into what calories mean for us in our everyday food and dietary choices. Let's face it, counting calories is probably the most mathematics people do after high school arithmetic! Almost every single packaged food product we buy at a grocery store—from a bag of nuts to a packet of chips to a bottle of herbs or spices—has a label with an estimate of calories it contains.

If you have ever been a calorie counter, chances are that you have memorized the basics: fats have nine calories per gram, while carbohydrates and proteins have four, and fibre has two. But the fact is that our sources of food are so varied and diverse that it is very difficult to work on the basis of averages. For example, the cells of different plants break down to different extents during the process of cooking. And the more broken down its cell walls are, the more access we have to the calories inside. Which is why our bodies don't extract all the calories contained in nuts and seeds— which are designed to resist digestion.

Our gut consists not only of the actual organs involved in digestion, but also the microbiota, as well as parts of the immune and nervous systems. And our gut responds differently to every kind of food it encounters. No wonder the phrase, 'You are what you eat', is so profound. For example, in some cases, where there might be potential pathogens in what we are consuming, our immune system might be activated to get involved. Or, in other cases, our bodies might need more heat energy to digest certain kinds of proteins, as compared to fats. But food labels don't really account for the energy or calories expended in these ways.

Calories in, calories out (CICO) used to be the mainstay of all diet plans, leading to the obsession with calorie counting. It was believed that weight gain or loss was simple arithmetic, involving the creation of a positive or negative calorie deficit. A rule of thumb was to create a 500-calorie deficit every day to lose a kilogram in two weeks. Although this sounds reasonable in theory, it is anything but that in practice. For the most part, calorie accounting is far too simplistic in its current model. We are better off focusing on balanced diets, working on hunger cues and limiting the number of times we eat in a day.

Empty calories are foods rich in calories but almost devoid of any real nutrition in the form of vitamins, minerals, fibre, essential fatty acids or other important nutrients. Think about the entire snack food industry that produces highly processed and industrialized food, high in salt, sugar and fat, engineered by high ranking scientists to entice your taste buds and leave you wanting more. If you look closely at the ad campaigns of many successful potato chip companies, you'll notice that they themselves highlight just how deliciously addictive their chips are—each crafted to perfection with the right amount of salt and fat, the perfect shape and texture and even the right colour to attack all our senses at once?

Most sodas and packaged foods that we consume are deprived of all nutritional value and pack just empty calories that may provide temporary energy spikes but do little to fuel our metabolism.

In the 2004 documentary *Super Size Me*, director Morgan Spurlock who, at thirty-two years of age, was fit and relatively healthy, decided to survive on nothing but food from fast food chain McDonald's for an entire month.[2] At the end of this thirty-day experiment, Spurlock had put on a whopping 11 kg, while his cholesterol had risen to 230 and he'd begun to suffer from heart palpitations and mood swings. If you were counting calories, you might get the right number from the meals at McDonald's, but almost all of those calories will be empty, high in salt, sugar and fat and containing almost nothing of any nutritious value.

Grains & Gluten

Recently, it seems, gluten intolerance has become rather common. But is there something more to it than the rage of gluten-free artisanal breads and pastas, or people self-diagnosing after hearing about Novak Djokovic and Gwyneth Paltrow going gluten-free? Many people wonder why we are suddenly discovering intolerances and allergies to something our human ancestors have been eating since the beginning of agriculture. But what they don't realize is that the grains we consume today are so different from the grains cultivated 10,000 years ago, that they may as well be completely different things. Not only have the grains been adapted and modified over the years, but we have also developed refining techniques to make them shinier, longer lasting and finer, processes that strip away much of their nutritional value. Modern manufacturing processes have created grains that have as much as forty times more gluten than grains cultivated even just a few decades ago.[3]

A study published in 2012 in the *Journal of Alzheimer's Disease* found that of the elderly people studied, those who consumed a diet high in carbohydrates were four times more likely than others to develop mild cognitive impairment, a precursor to Alzheimer's.[4] The carbohydrates we consume in the form of grains cause inflammation that is also linked to neurological conditions such as anxiety, depression and ADHD.

The good news is that if you love your grains, there are options. If you think you might have a mild gluten sensitivity, try cutting all wheat and wheat products from your diet. Barley and rye also contain gluten, as do some packaged forms of oats. Instead, pick from a variety of wholesome gluten-free grains, and if you can, try to find less processed and refined versions. For example, red or brown rice is rich in fibre, filling and tasty. Millets are also a great option for people looking at grain alternatives, as are quinoa, buckwheat flour and sorghum.

Chances are, you are not gluten sensitive, especially if you are from a culture that has historically consumed wheat. But if you have persistent bowel issues, you might want to get tested for gluten sensitivity. If you are intolerant or sensitive, going gluten-free will do wonders for your health. Even if you are not, making wheat just one of many grains in a diverse diet is a good idea. My own diet has recently shifted to include more ragi and other millets, and I find myself enjoying the taste of these far more than I once enjoyed wheat.

THE DAIRY DILEMMA

In India, dairy is a big part of our dietary culture. It is an essential ingredient in many of our favourite dishes, from butter chicken to payasam. In addition, most of us grew up drinking (or being forced to drink) large glasses of milk at least once, if not twice, a day. Milk has therefore also been an important source of protein for many people in India, particularly vegetarians.

Lactose intolerance is the inability to digest lactose, the sugar present in milk and dairy products (other than curd and paneer, in which most lactose is broken down by fermentation). This is because most humans stop producing lactase, the enzyme required to break down lactose, after childhood. Lactase persistence has been discovered in some populations, however, allowing them to continue consuming milk as adults. Most of us in India presume we have lactase persistence, but recent studies have found that this isn't true. Despite our long history of raising cattle and consuming milk in various forms, it turns out that, according to some studies, over 60 per cent of Indians are lactose intolerant. One 1981 study found that lactose intolerance might be more prevalent in south India than in the north.

A lactose intolerance might not always present itself as a violent reaction to any consumption of dairy. It might result in mild discomfort or other digestion-related symptoms that you usually ignore. If you suspect that dairy is not your best friend, observe how you feel when you reduce or cut it out completely. Many people discover they feel great when they remove dairy from their diet. The only thing to keep in mind is that if milk was a main source of protein for you, ensure you find other sources. Fortunately, if you miss milk in your tea or coffee, you can now choose from many vegan alternatives such as oat or almond milk.

MAKING FATS WORK

We evolved to crave fats—an integral component of a healthy diet—primarily because of their caloric density. Not only do we get more than twice the number of calories from a gram of fat than we do from carbs, but fats are digested far slower, providing energy for longer periods. This is probably why we originally started putting ghee on our rice and rotis as a staple ritual in most Indian households, or buttering bread in other parts of the world. As fats started to get vilified, however, out went this habit, thus depriving us not only of a cultural connection, but also of an excellent source of nutrition.

The misadventures of fats lasted almost two generations, starting in the 1960s and finally coming full circle by around 2010. Now, thanks to better nutrition science as well as the advocacy of self-styled health gurus, we know exactly what's going on with fats and how to make them work for us. Here are a few basic rules to keep in mind:

1. Monounsaturated fats, which tend to be liquid at room temperature, are quite good for us. Some sources of these include avocados, almonds, cashews, olive oil and sesame oil, among others.
2. Polyunsaturated fats are considered particularly healthy for us and are found in walnuts, flaxseed, fish oil, sunflower seeds and various other seeds.
3. Saturated fats fought a valiant battle on our behalf and now stand vindicated. Most dairy fats, coconut oil, cheese, palm oil and many animal fats are saturated fats. These are usually solid at room temperature. Saturated fats in moderate quantities are good and can even help raise good cholesterol in the body.
4. The worst kind of fats are trans fats and you should avoid these like the plague. Trans fats don't occur in nature and are usually produced at high temperatures. Most junk foods are laden with trans fats, a result of the process of deep frying, and should be avoided.

As you plan your plate, pay attention to whether there are enough fats in your meal and also to the kinds of fats you are using. We now have many options to choose from to make our meals more tasty and more nutritious. The only thing to watch out for is quantity because fats pack quite a punch in terms of calorific value. Adding a small amount of fat to each meal will also help you get better at using stored body fats for energy, which is critical for healthy metabolism.

HEALTH HACK #8: A Dollop of Ghee

An all-natural ingredient that is an integral part of an Indian kitchen, ghee is a healthy source of fat, with antioxidant properties, containing several fat-soluble vitamins. Our Indian ancestors recognized this nutritional powerhouse, adding it to almost every meal and including it in treatments for overall health.

DEALING WITH SUGAR

You might have heard the phrase, 'sugar is the new tobacco', and while this might not be factually accurate, it definitely draws attention to the hidden dangers of sugar. Like fat—and perhaps even more so—we evolved to crave sugar.

We find sweetened food and drink irresistible; the more we consume, the more we desire it. Sugar, it seems, is addictive. Because it was such a rare source of immediate energy whenever we could find it, we have evolved to greet sugar consumption with a dopamine kick, which makes us feel very good. In the past it encouraged us to gorge on fruits so that we could pack all that extra energy for a rainy day, but in modern times it has turned us into addicts who proudly refer to our 'sweet tooth' almost as if it were a badge of honour or an endearing personality quirk. It is a classic case of a nifty survival mechanism gone haywire with the modern lifestyle, masterfully exploited by industrial food complexes.

One of the earliest research studies that looked at food cravings was published in 1976 by Anthony Sclafani and is considered seminal in the field.[5] While an assistant professor of psychology at Brooklyn College, Sclafani needed to fatten up some rats for a study. However, on their usual diet of dog food, they just didn't put on enough weight. Remembering a time as a graduate student, when he discovered how much rats loved Froot Loops® the sickly sweet breakfast cereal that kids love, Sclafani began feeding this group of rats cookies, candy and other sugary snacks and desserts. After just a few weeks on this sweet diet, they grew obese. The rats began to crave sugar so much, that their desire won over all biological signals to stop eating. This is the study that led to many others that revealed the link between sugar and compulsive overeating—including one in which rats continued to eat cheesecake even after they were conditioned to expect an electrical shock when they did.

How our bodies digest sugar also gives us insight into what exactly it does to our health. Monosaccharides are simple sugars composed of single molecules, and include glucose, galactose and fructose, the latter found in honey and fruit.[6] Complex sugars or disaccharides are formed of two sugar molecules—the most common of these is sucrose, extracted from sugarcane and beets, composed of one molecule of fructose and one of glucose. Lactose is a complex sugar found in milk. High-fructose corn syrup, one of the cheapest and most common sources of sugar used in recent times, is the result of corn being broken down into glucose molecules, half of which are then chemically transformed into fructose.

Despite what many might believe, the body cannot tell the difference between naturally occurring and processed sugars. However, it can only absorb sugars in monosaccharide form. During digestion, disaccharides are broken down into their individual molecules. While glucose is managed by insulin, fructose is digested by the liver, releasing fat molecules as a by-product. Fructose is added to processed food and beverages in large quantities, which can eventually overwhelm the liver. In addition, fructose, unlike glucose, does not suppress appetite, often leading to overeating.

Perhaps the biggest problem with sugar is that cutting it out is not just about giving up desserts or drinking tea and coffee without adding sugar, because there are hidden sugars almost everywhere. From ketchup and other readymade sauces and condiments, to fried savoury snacks, even the most unsuspecting packaged food item on our shelves is loaded with sugars.

Fruit is probably the safest form of sugar we consume because it comes naturally combined with fibres, vitamins, minerals and phytochemicals that are good for us. It thus takes us longer to metabolize these as compared to processed sugars. For many years, fruit juices were touted as good for health, but the fact is that these strip the fruits of their fibre leaving mostly sugar in your glass. A few servings of fruit a day can be both delicious and beneficial, but too many sugary fruits can have adverse health effects.

The Question of Alcohol

Alcohol is technically the fourth macronutrient, containing 7 calories per gram, but since it is not essential to our survival, we don't mention it while talking about the main macros. The truth is, we're better off without alcohol in our diets. I don't mean to be a party pooper, especially for those who enjoy a few glasses on a weekend, but in a book about health, we cannot ignore its ill effects. There was a time when it was considered not just okay but actually beneficial to have a drink or two every now and then. More recently, many of us have delighted in the research about the health and supposed longevity benefits of red wine. Unfortunately, much of this research is still controversial, and to actually gain the anti-ageing benefits of resveratrol, we'd need to consume something like three litres of wine a day!

On the other hand, regular alcohol consumption can cause liver and pancreatic damage, raise blood pressure, increase the risk for heart attacks and even cause early-onset Alzheimer's. Alcohol is also associated with many types of cancer. If I'm being really honest, alcohol has no nutritional value and does more harm than good. When we drink, our satiety hormones might get suppressed, leading us to crave unhealthy food and gain weight. Alcohol is dehydrating, aggravates our stomach lining and prevents us from getting a good night's rest as it interferes with the REM phase of sleep. Women also tend to be more susceptible to the damage caused by alcohol.

Unfortunately, alcohol has become a big part of our culture—something we associate with unwinding after a stressful day of work and celebrating with family and friends. And while I won't tell you that you absolutely cannot have that glass of red wine at a friend's farewell, I also won't tell you that a few drinks now and then are good for your health. Because, let's face it, they just aren't.

HEALTH HACK #9: Microbiome Testing

A microbiome test will profile the genetic sequence of all the microorganisms in your gut, giving you a picture of the good inhabitants and the not so good guys, and their diversity. This can help diagnose any chronic conditions, and could also be useful in determining whether you need to supplement with probiotics, and tailoring your diet to the needs of your gut flora.

Gut—Your Second Brain

Tell me what you eat, I'll tell you who you are.—Anthelme
Brillat-Savarin

Our gut and stomach in general have been a fertile source of
jokes for comedians—what with the variety of sounds and smells
and politically incorrect references that involve the gut in one
way or another. Unlike children who have no inhibitions, we
generally prefer our guts to stay out of sight, out of mind and out
of our hearing! Some find it funny; others find it embarrassing
or disgusting, but for scientists who want to learn about health
in earnest, the working of the gut is one of the most fascinating
areas of health research. The more we learn about this system,
the more we discover about the extraordinary role played by the
gut to keep us in the pink of health, occasional sounds and smells
notwithstanding!

Recent research has shed light on the intimate connection
between the brain and the gut, which is now being called 'the
second brain'. In this context, the ideas of having 'butterflies
in your stomach' or having 'a gut feeling' take on entirely new
and profound meanings. So does the phrase, 'You are what
you eat.' Our diet and our digestion affect our moods, and our
moods affect the way we eat or what we choose to eat. Have
you ever noticed how stress makes you overeat or how eating
certain kinds of food gives you a sense of emotional comfort
or discomfort? And what about that Sunday brunch-induced
food coma? This field of research is one of the most fascinating,
as studies reveal the depth and intricacy of the brain-gut
connection.

When you think of the gut, you might often visualize just the digestive tract. However, the gut is a complex system that includes not only this tract, but also the intestinal flora or the microorganisms of the gut, as well as the nervous and immune systems located within and around the walls of the intestines. In fact, about two-thirds of the body's entire immune system resides in the gut, protected by a fragile, single-cell layer lining. The longest cranial nerve, the vagus nerve, originates in the brain stem and connects to the abdomen.

The digestive system begins in the mouth which has more nerve endings than most other parts of the body. After being chewed and swallowed, the food we eat ends up in the stomach where it is treated to acids and enzymes that begin the actual digestive process. From here, it travels to the small intestine. In order to ensure that we were able to absorb as many nutrients as possible from our food, evolution ensured that our small intestines have a huge surface area, covered with tiny protruding finger-like forms called villi and microvilli. The pancreas and liver secrete enzymes that act on the partially digested food in the small intestine, along with a range of bacteria. But the large intestine or colon is where most of the microbes of the gut reside, where they survive on the leftovers of our food, breaking them down and absorbing nutrients that our bodies would not otherwise be able to. The leftovers of the leftovers—or the food substances and particles that the bacteria don't consume—are excreted twenty-four to seventy-two hours after a meal. Almost half of excreted stool is composed of bacteria, dead and alive.

The bacteria in the gut multiply at a great pace, and can double their numbers every thirty or forty minutes. Despite the fact that we haven't treated these inhabitants of our bodies very well in the last few decades—drastically changing our diets from those of our hunter–gatherer ancestors—the microbiota have survived thanks to their incredible plasticity. They might be able to adapt, but the fact is that, antibiotic use, diets low in diversity and the empty-calorie fast foods we consume constantly change the diversity, species and resilience of our gut flora. Of course, there are harmful bacteria too—like salmonella or vibrio cholera. These pathogens are what led to the development of antibiotics which, unfortunately, have started destroying the good bacteria in our bodies.

If you still think that tiny, almost-invisible microorganisms cannot be that important in the health of the body, here's a fascinating experiment that might change your mind. In their book, *The Good Gut: Taking Care of Your Weight, Your Mood and Your Long-Term Health*, Justin and Erica Sonnenberg describe the lab of their mentor Dr Jeffrey Gordon, a gastroenterologist and microbiome scientist.[7] Here, he keeps a collection of gnotobiotic mice—mice, in whose guts every microorganism has been identified and can be colonized by a human microbiota. The lab has demonstrated that just by altering the microbiota of these mice, they can induce the mice to become obese or lean without changing any other aspect of diet or lifestyle. This study highlights the critical role that gut bacteria play in our pursuit of health, emphasizing the fact that we just cannot ignore our gut.

Transferring Gut Bugs

Despite knowing just how profoundly the microorganisms of our gut affect every single aspect of our health and our lives, some of the research into the gut still sounds bizarre, even pretty gross. One of these ideas that is still being researched is that of a microbiome transplant, which is essentially the transfer of microorganisms from the gut of a healthy individual into the gut of someone facing specific health problems. This is usually done through the transfer of faecal matter via pills (or another less pleasant route) to address things like obesity and metabolic syndrome. While research into this procedure is still ongoing, there is evidence to show that it might actually work!

The enteric nervous system, often called the 'second brain', controls our body's digestion through a network of over 100 million nerves and chemicals that communicate with the central nervous system. Once we decide what to eat and eat it—whether we cook our meals, choose off a fancy five-star cafe menu, or order in through one of several food delivery apps so that we can eat and watch Netflix at the same time—the rest of the process of digestion is unconscious. This is one of the most unique aspects of digestion, that it is controlled largely by the autonomic nervous system and happens out of sight, out of mind.

The signals from the enteric nervous system seem to be connected to the regions of the brain responsible for things like self-awareness, emotion, morality, fear, memory and motivation. The vagus nerve connects the digestive system to the brain, and studies on humans have found that by stimulating this nerve at different frequencies, people can be made to feel emotions like comfort or anxiety. Once we understand the deep connection that the gut has with the brain, it becomes easy to see why we have such a complicated emotional relationship with food. Our guts are in continuous communication with our brains and what we eat has a direct impact on our mood and emotions. In fact, research now suggests that probiotics—which contain healthy bacteria to restore the gut flora—can have a positive impact on depression and anxiety.[8]

To understand just how intimately linked our guts and brains are, you should know that 90 per cent of the serotonin in our bodies is produced in the gut. Serotonin is one of the most important neurotransmitters in regulating mood, memory, sleep, social connections and, of course, digestion. You could also look at a baby, whose entire life seems to revolve around its gut—needing to be constantly fed, burped, or have its nappy changed! A baby's emotions are also closely linked to hunger and satiety, and even as adults we feel 'hangry'—a millennial term coined to express the irritability and moodiness we experience when we don't get fed on time! It isn't so far-fetched then, to say that our gut is probably affecting our moods through our days and lives.

One of the most commonly discussed factors in gut-brain studies is stress. When the brain encounters stress, it requires extra energy to deal with the situation or pressure; energy that it borrows from the gut at the cost of smooth digestion. If temporary, this situation isn't particularly harmful, but when stress is chronic, it can cause long-term and painful complications. The gut receives less blood, and the mucus in the gut wall gets thinner. Immunity can get affected, and all of this could lead to inflammation. Some theories say that this state of stress changes the collection of bacteria in the gut—those that can withstand the new environment survive, while others don't.

The numerous species of microbes within us each have their own genome, and together, all the genes of all the microbes in our bodies, is called the microbiome. In a way, just like your own genetic code, your microbiome is what makes you, you. In 2007, soon after the Human Genome Project was completed, the Human Microbiome Project was launched. This project was based on the understanding that the genomes of the microbes that inhabit the human body carried out processes that the human body wouldn't need to evolve to do on its own. It aimed to use the technology from the Human Genome Project to characterize the genetic material of the body's microbes. This, it was hoped, would open up more avenues for personalized medicine and healthcare, as well as early disease diagnosis and prevention.

The microbes in the human body of 2023 are probably so different from those of our palaeolithic ancestors that the two groups would barely recognize each other! In fact, the microbiota of a modern human is probably woefully unhealthy, thanks to our urban lifestyles and diets. In order to understand what an actual, healthy and functioning microbiota looks like, the best samples are those of the Hadza tribe.[9] They are among the last populations who still follow the hunter–gatherer way of life completely, living in the Great Rift Valley of Tanzania—an area, incidentally, that has some of the oldest remains of our human ancestors. Living on a diet that is far from agriculture and antibiotic-injected meat, the Hadza hunt their own meat, and gather their own berries, fruit, seeds, honey and tubers. They consume approximately 100–150 g of fibre per day, which is almost ten times that consumed by the average Indian. It's no surprise then, that the Hadza have far more diverse microbes living inside of them than any of us do today. It appears that the greater the processed foods in one's diet and the more often one has been prescribed antibiotics, the less diverse one's gut microbes. And diversity is what protects us from completely collapsing at the first sign of infection.

Probiotics are non-pathogenic, beneficial microorganisms that include bacteria and yeast used to treat gastrointestinal disorders. It is believed that probiotics, after being ingested orally, attach to the lining of the intestines to prevent pathogenic bacteria from causing harm. Some types produce lactic acid and other compounds that inhibit the growth of harmful microorganisms. Overall, they can help restore the balance and health of the gut, replacing microorganisms that might have been destroyed by a course of antibiotics or by an unhealthy diet. In addition to treating diarrhoea, irritable bowel syndrome, and other gastrointestinal problems, probiotics have also proved to be effective at treating eczema and are being studied for their use in the treatment of mental health illnesses as well as diabetes and obesity.

While looking for a probiotic supplement, try and keep a few things in mind. Since every single one of us has a unique microbiome, generalized commercial-use probiotics might not necessarily be perfectly suited to your gut. There are also some foods that are good sources of probiotics, such as yoghurt, buttermilk, cheese and, in India, fermented foods like pickles, idli and dosa. The common international sources of probiotics are tempeh, sauerkraut, kimchi, miso and blue cheese, among many others. In addition, instead of just focusing on probiotic sources of food, remember that having a healthy gut flora in the first place is important, and this can be maintained with a diet rich in antioxidants and fibre.

So, what can we do to keep our guts healthy? If you want to have the dirty details of your gut bacteria, you could do an at-home stool test with one of the several companies offering microbiome testing. With an understanding of our microbiome, we can make much better choices about our diet and lifestyle. In general, eating a diet low in processed and sugary foods but rich in raw foods, diversified and local ingredients, fermented foods, as well as ensuring you consume some fruit or vegetables with their skin intact can help to keep the gut in good shape. If you often take antibiotics, this will have a significant adverse effect on the gut. If you find that certain foods like processed carbs or dairy products leave you feeling uneasy or fatigued, try to remove them from your diet. The other thing is to pay attention to how you design mealtimes at your home. Make sure you don't have the TV blaring in the background and avoid stressful dinner table conversations. Eating should be a joyful and pleasant time, where you are present in the moment, experiencing the flavours and textures of food slowly and with mindfulness. Taking care of chronic stress can also help cheer up the microorganisms in your gut.

Hopefully, armed with this bit of nutrition science, you can make better food choices in your everyday life—adding good fats to your diet, taking better care of your gut and its inhabitants, fasting occasionally and treating sugar with a substantial amount of scepticism.

THE CAVEMAN DIET

The caveman or paleo diet is based on the idea that humans are genetically programmed for a certain kind of diet and lifestyle— that of our hunter–gatherer ancestors. We spent most of our ancient past in the Palaeolithic Age, a period of almost 2.5 million years that led to the evolution of the human species as we now know it. However, with the agricultural revolution about 10,000 years ago, followed by the industrial revolution about 200 years ago, we have abandoned that lifestyle completely. We've gone from spending most of our days on our feet—hunting, foraging for food, finding safety, chasing prey—to spending most of our days sitting. Squinting at a screen. Slouching over a desk. And eating things out of packets that don't even slightly resemble the foods of our ancestors. This mismatch has resulted in what are aptly called the diseases of civilization, from diabetes and cancer, to hypertension and heart disease. The paleo diet, therefore, advises a return to the eating habits of our Palaeolithic ancestors.

If ancient humans were eating wild berries and tubers, those fruits and vegetables are likely to be good for us. If they were not munching on lab-designed deep-fried potato snacks, those snacks are probably best avoided by us too. If our ancestors were content having one or two meals a day, that's a good idea for us. If they were not plotting a late-night dessert raid on the fridge, midnight feasts are probably not a good idea for us either. It is as simple as that.

A paleo diet usually consists of meat, fish and vegetables, minimally cooked using natural fats like butter and olive oil. Those following this way of life are encouraged to eat grass-fed or free-range poultry, meat and fish, and wild herbs and plants that are seasonal and fresh. Usually not on the menu are cereal grains including wheat, corn and rice, as well as pasteurized dairy products. While there is some debate about what exactly our Palaeolithic ancestors ate, and about different interpretations of the Paleo lifestyle, the best part about this diet is that it focuses on whole, seasonal, unprocessed and unrefined foods—and if you ask me, that sounds like the ideal kind of diet.

Plant-Based Diets

Despite its title, this section is by no means an indictment of animal protein, which, for many reasons, is an excellent food choice for many. Ideally, animal-based protein should be antibiotic-free, free range and naturally sourced which, unfortunately, is not always the case with most meat products today. Even if you can find clean and healthy meat, some moderation is probably the best way to go. After all, that's how humans ate in the wild. They mostly foraged for food and ate what grew on trees, only occasionally enjoying a feast after a successful hunt. In fact, as an interesting aside, if humans needed meat to survive, the population of our species would never have reached the numbers it has. The population of purely meat-eating predators tends to be very small in the jungle.

Plant-based food is an excellent source of fibre, antioxidants, and, contrary to popular belief, can also provide the protein we need to stay in good health. A plant-based diet usually consists of plenty of vegetables, both raw and cooked, fruits, beans, pulses and lentils, as well as seeds and nuts in smaller quantities.

Over the years, the evidence in favour of a plant-based diet has stacked up. It is found to be one of the most effective diets for weight-management and the reversal of obesity.[10] Studies have also discovered that the prevalence of heart disease, high blood pressure, diabetes and obesity is lower in vegetarian populations. A plant-based diet is associated with reduced insulin resistance, and therefore, may help in the treatment or prevention of diabetes.

If you are considering a shift to a plant-based diet, remember this way of eating doesn't mean you blindly eat any and all non-animal foods in a random and unplanned way. To get all the essential nutrients for your body, you need to make sure your diet is well-balanced. You should also be aware that you might need to supplement with or look out for plant-based sources of calcium, vitamin B12, essential fatty acids and iron which are easier to find in a non-vegetarian diet.

It is also a good idea to try to eliminate or at least drastically reduce the consumption of processed foods. If you want to take things slow, just begin to cut down on your meat intake. You might want to continue consuming some dairy products, or you might find great alternatives to the things you love. At the end of the day, it is also about how you feel—whether you have enough physical and mental energy every day, whether you feel satiated after a meal and whether you truly enjoy what you eat.

TO KETO OR NOT TO KETO

Every few years, a new fad takes the world of food by storm. If a typical fad is a storm, the surge of keto is nothing less than a gale force hurricane.

Keto diets work by getting the body into a state of ketosis, in which fat becomes the primary source of fuel. This requires you to eliminate or drastically reduce the carbohydrates in your diet. Typically, in a keto diet, you get 65 per cent of your calories from fat, 25 per cent from protein and less than 10 per cent from carbohydrates, which amounts to about 50 g or the equivalent of four slices of bread per day. When your diet consists of mostly fat, your body feels as though it is in a permanent fasting state without actually fasting, triggering survival circuits. This improves fat metabolism so much that the body is able to gain its energy from stored fat as efficiently as it does from dietary fat, which is great for health as well as weight loss.

Ketogenic diets were first used in the 1920s to treat epilepsy by keeping patients on extended fasts of up to twenty days with a diet mostly consisting of MCT (medium chain triglyceride) oil. In the 1960s, scientists noted that MCTs significantly improved fat metabolism compared to ordinary fat sources.

According to some theories, our palaeolithic ancestors probably spent a large part of their existence in ketosis, especially during periods of food scarcity when they drew on stored fat for energy. More recently, studies have found that the Inuit were probably permanently in a ketogenic state thanks to their traditional diet that consisted largely of fatty meat and fish.

Before you start a keto diet, make sure to do your research. Figure out your meal plans and find the best local and seasonal sources of healthy fats and proteins. Again, you might want to very slowly start reducing the quantity of carbohydrates you eat each day and see how this makes you feel. It's also a good idea to speak to your doctor or nutritionist before going all the way, especially if you are diabetic or have any other health conditions. Important to note is the fact that the keto diet relies quite heavily on animal protein. It is possible to go keto as a vegetarian, but not only might this be harder, but could also come with the risk of developing nutritional deficiencies. Biohacker Dave Asprey recommends cyclic ketosis, alternating between a no-carb keto diet, a moderate carb diet and fasting days. In this way, the body learns to shift between sugar and fat as sources of fuel, maintaining what Asprey calls metabolic flexibility. This might be a good way to see if the keto diet works for you, observing the response of your body and mind.

INTERMITTENT FASTING

The humans of the past knew intuitively what science has now incontrovertibly established. Fasting is good for us. Period. Fasting has a rich history and is also steeped in many of the world's religions. From Hippocrates and Aristotle to Benjamin Franklin, some of the best minds of history have believed that fasting is an important aspect of good health. The practice of fasting is also woven into many faiths.

The world record for the longest fast is held by Angus Barbieri who went without food for a year and seventeen days. A Scotsman, Barbieri weighed 207 kg at the age of twenty-seven. His doctors recommended a short fast to address his obesity, and, finding that he was managing quite well without food, he decided to keep going. He ended up fasting for 382 days, surviving on just black tea, black coffee and sparkling water, with multivitamins and supplements to ensure essential nutrients. He went to the hospital for regular checkups and doctors found that his body was functioning perfectly well on his extended fast. Barbieri finally broke his fast (with a boiled egg, bread and butter, for those who are curious) when he reached his goal weight of 82 kg, having shed a whopping 125 kg. While Barbieri's fast was extreme, he did manage to maintain his new weight, and the story proved that humans can go fairly long periods without food.

What this means is that our bodies are not only very strongly shaped by fasting but are adapted to survive and thrive in starvation mode. Intermittent Fasting (IF) hacks into this ancient code by mimicking the way humans always ate, which is infrequently. Intermittent fasting isn't so much a diet as an eating pattern, involving periods of fasting and periods of 'feeding'. A typical pattern prescribes a short eating window of 6–10 hours in which you get all your calories, and after which, you don't eat. This means fasting for fourteen hours (mild IF) to eighteen hours (serious IF!). The upshot of an IF diet is that you can eat whatever you want, as long as it is not atrocious junk food. Maintaining a healthy carb, fat and protein ratio in an IF diet will still give you the full benefit of fasting without creating a state of severe starvation that a keto diet gone wrong can lead to. My own experience has convinced me of the great benefits of IF, but recent research[11] claims there is no significant difference between IF and daily caloric restriction without time restriction when it comes to reduction in weight, fat and risk for metabolic disease. I believe that reducing calories without reducing the frequency of eating doesn't give the body the time it needs to get into ketosis, so I'm going to stay tuned for more exciting studies that are sure to come from the field.

SHARING A TABLE WITH A TAPEWORM

Strange as it may sound, Victorian women aspired for a beauty ideal inspired by patients of tuberculosis—pale skin, pink cheeks, rosy lips and, most importantly, a frail figure. In pursuit of this bizarre standard of beauty, they pursued equally bizarre practices including the tapeworm diet. Doctors would prescribe pills containing tapeworm eggs that would hatch inside the body of a woman, consuming a part of whatever the woman was eating. This would allow her to stay skinny without actually going hungry. Removing the tapeworm was an altogether nastier business which I won't get into here, but the most surprising thing, however, might be the fact that this diet is said to have outlasted the Victorians!

Apart from a daily fasting schedule, many people also choose to do a complete twenty-four-hour fast on one or two days of the week. Others do a twenty-four-hour fast every alternate weekday. Another form of intermittent fasting is known as the 5:2 diet— featuring five days of normal eating and two days of restricting calories to 500–600 per day. And finally, skipping the occasional meal or making breakfast optional are also simple forms of intermittent fasting.

Given that intermittent fasting as an eating plan does not specify what kinds of food to include in your meals, you might want to try and follow a balanced diet of plant-based whole foods as much as you can. This kind of plan is also easy to experiment with and adapt to suit your needs. However, do check in with your doctor before you try any form of fasting, especially if you are on any medication or have elevated levels of blood sugar.

HOW TO GET FASTING

1. Choose a fasting window that works for you. This could be as short as twelve hours and as long as eighteen hours. It could be fasting for four or five days a week or going on longer fasts less frequently.

2. Increasing the fasting window can be hard, so start very slow, first postponing breakfast by an hour. Give yourself two to three days to adjust to every increase in hours of fasting, taking two to three weeks to get from eleven to sixteen hours.

3. Listen to your body and observe how you feel as you gradually increase the fasting window. Give yourself time and don't do anything that makes you feel stressed or uncomfortable.

4. Stay hydrated by consuming as many zero-calorie fluids as you can, including water, black coffee or tea and even water with lemon and salt as an electrolyte drink.

5. As your body adapts to longer hours of fasting, you might notice that you are more energetic and that your mind is sharper. The evolutionary theory for this is that the energy saved on digestion was used to sharpen focus for a hunt.

6. Try to follow a 'no eating after dark' rule: this will help you sleep better, and a good night's rest will help you extend your fasting period in the morning.

7. You might find that the best time to exercise is at the end of a fast, after which you can break the fast with a healthy meal containing protein and fat to keep you full.

8. Be flexible—take a break from IF once in a while, change up your fasting windows or experiment with a twenty-four-hour fast, depending on what suits your current lifestyle.

9. Use your fasting experiments to get in touch with your true hunger cues—ask yourself if you are actually hungry, if you are just habituated to eating at a certain time or if you are craving something which is very different from real hunger.

10. Women with PCOS or those who are on their menstrual cycle, trying to conceive or going through menopause should always consult a doctor before any kind of fasting.

LOCAL FOODS

With globalization and the industrialization of food, it has become possible to eat almost every kind of fruit, vegetable and grain from every part of the world, even out of season and thousands of miles away from where it is grown.

In truth, the seasonal availability of different produce, and indigenous varieties of crops that grow in specific landscapes and climates are important ways of ensuring diversity in our diets and all-round wellness through nutrition. When we consume the same produce throughout the year, in summer and winter, we become more vulnerable to food allergies and intolerances.

Eating out of season also means that the produce on our plates has been transported over huge distances or been stored for a long time, and is therefore unlikely to be very fresh. It's possible that it has also been grown with the use of a lot of chemical input or been artificially ripened. As a result, in addition to the carbon footprint and environmental costs of this transport, we're probably not even getting all the nutrients we think we are when we eat kiwis from New Zealand, guavas from Thailand or kale from the US while sitting in Bangalore!

Fortunately, eating local is 'in' again. It is also accessible, whether you decide to shop at your local fruit and vegetable vendor who doesn't have a cold storage unit—meaning she has only fresh and seasonal produce—or at a neighbourhood organic store, farmer's market or even online.

Detoxing

Detoxification is the elimination of toxins from the body to promote wellness or weight loss through a combination of lifestyle and diet plans. There are many ways in which you can detox—from juice cleanses to luxurious wellness spa experiences, or just adding supplements or removing fast foods from your diet. A detox might also involve slightly more intense methods such as the use of laxatives or enemas to flush out the system. The central idea is to remove toxins that our modern lifestyles expose us to.

There are several detox diets on the market, but the problem is that many of these commercial ventures, that sell a product or supplement of their own, do not really have your best interests in mind. In fact, there are some who believe that the entire concept of a detox is nothing but a glorified marketing pitch, with no basis in science. It offers people a quick fix to absolve themselves of the guilt associated with their unhealthy lifestyles of binge eating, binge drinking, and binge-watching Netflix, with no exercise whatsoever. Several of the detox products on the market, from pills and juices to supposedly miracle powders and smoothies, do not stand up to the rigours of scientific testing, and often, the manufacturers themselves have no idea what the 'toxins' they claim to cleanse actually are.[12]

The idea of a detox in itself, however, isn't a bad one. Often, in our normal routine of everyday life, we don't pay enough attention to the way we are eating, living, sleeping or moving. A detox is like a gentle pause button that slows you down and allows you to take stock of what your health goals are and how to reach them. Keeping this in mind, and after consultation with your doctor, you might want to try your own version of a detox. This might be as simple as limiting how often you eat out to just once or twice a week or eating your favourite dessert only on the weekend.

Your body has a highly sophisticated detoxification system in place already, involving the liver, kidneys, gastrointestinal system, skin and lungs. However, we are now exposed to a whole host of toxins that our bodies did not evolve to handle, which is why we might need to give it a hand every once in a while. You might choose different ways of detoxing—a period of total fasting, a liquid-only cleanse or even just taking a break from certain things like sugar, dairy, meat or processed carbs and packaged foods. Whichever form and duration of detoxing you choose, there are a few general things you should keep in mind.

Drinking lots of water is a great way of constantly flushing out toxins while staying hydrated. Taking a steam bath or going to a sauna can also speed up the release of toxins, as can sweating through physical activity and exercise. And of course, ensuring you get enough rest and sleep ensures that your body has time to fix itself and the energy to keep you going. It's important to note that extreme forms of starvation or supplementation can have powerful negative health effects, and moderation, like always, might be the way to go.

In Summary

Keep in Mind

1. The modern diet is convenient, affordable and accessible, but includes pre-packaged, oily, deep-fried and sugary products that wreak havoc on health.
2. A healthy diet has a balanced mix of macronutrients—carbohydrates, fats and protein.
3. While most diets are based on calorie counting and the calories-in, calories-out theory, food is more than just calories. Most junk foods are considered empty calories as they are high in calories but almost devoid of nutrition.
4. Techniques of refining grains may have made us more gluten-intolerant and studies have linked gluten to conditions such as Alzheimer's.
5. A surprisingly high number of Indian adults are likely to be lactose intolerant, despite arguments about the cultural history of milk.
6. While most fats are good for us, trans fats—or those produced through high temperatures like deep frying—should be avoided at all costs.
7. Sugar is addictive and does not offer any nutritional benefits. Aside from a few servings of fruit per day, it is best to avoid added sugars, fruit juices and artificial sweeteners.
8. Alcohol causes liver damage, raises blood pressure, increases risk for heart attack and some cancers, interferes with sleep, dehydrates us and makes us crave unhealthy food.
9. Our guts are intimately linked to our brains and overall health, including immunity and mental health, and it will serve us well to support the diversity of its microorganisms.

10. The Paleo diet mimics that of our hunter–gatherer ancestors, including meat, vegetables, nuts and seeds, with no artificial sugars, dairy or refined food products.

11. Plant-based diets, rich in fibre and antioxidants, have been found to be effective in weight loss, reversing diabetes and lowering insulin resistance.

12. The keto diet requires getting 65 per cent of your daily calories from fat, 25 per cent from proteins and 10 per cent from carbohydrates, so the body switches to burning fat as fuel, the state of ketosis.

13. Intermittent fasting is designed to give the body a rest by extending the fasting window up to twelve or sixteen hours, regulating sugar metabolism and helping in weight loss.

14. The seasonal availability of local foods supports a fresh, diverse and healthy diet.

15. While many commercial detoxes are simply marketing gimmicks, the idea of detoxing the body is like a gentle pause button to refresh your eating habits.

Take Action

1. Plan your meals once a week and go grocery shopping, so that you aren't forced to choose pre-packaged food products which might be more convenient.

2. Pick unprocessed and unrefined carbs when possible and add healthy fats and protein to meals—especially breakfast and snacks—to keep you feeling full for longer.

3. Don't get too caught up in calorie counting and focus more on quality than quantity.

4. Ensure wheat is just one of an array of diverse grains on your plate—include red and brown rice, millets and more. And if

you think gluten doesn't suit you, try reducing wheat or get tested for gluten sensitivity.

5. If you suspect dairy is causing you trouble, reduce it or cut it out. Find alternatives like oat or almond milk, but make sure you're still getting enough protein in your diet.

6. Add good fats like yoghurt or coconut oil to your breakfasts and snacks, so that you aren't grazing all day.

7. Avoid sugar as far as possible, including fruit juices and artificial sweeteners. A few servings of fruit a day, on the other hand, has its benefits.

8. If good health is your goal, alcohol simply cannot be a part of your daily or weekly routine. An occasional glass on a special occasion is the way to go.

9. Choose probiotic supplements that aren't loaded with sugar, and try to add probiotic foods to your diet, such as buttermilk, pickles, idli and dosa, kimchi and miso.

10. Even if you are non-vegetarian, make sure to have several servings of vegetables and greens with every meal.

11. Check in with your doctor before trying a keto diet and, once you start, observe the effects not just on your body but also on your mind—focus and productivity.

12. Start intermittent fasting by postponing breakfast by an hour every few days, and see how you feel. Take it slow, and speak to a doctor first!

13. For your weekly shopping, find a neighbourhood fruit and vegetable vendor who doesn't have a refrigerator—this means everything is super fresh and local.

14. If you're trying a detox, first check in with your doctor, remember to stay hydrated and don't do anything extreme without a professional to guide you.

4

FITNESS & RECOVERY

The definition of a really good workout: when you hate doing it, but you love finishing it.—Anonymous

It can be argued that the entire enterprise of industrialization over the last 300 years has been devoted to inventing every possible type of labour-saving device so that we don't need to move a muscle to do a thing. It may be hard to imagine that we used to do everything by hand and on our feet for our entire evolutionary history, until just a few hundred years ago. It has been argued in biological sciences that brains primarily evolved for locomotion. Our brain processes all five senses to gauge where the food sources are and where the possible dangers may be so that we can go where the food is and run away from danger. The brain would process incoming signals, make quick calculations and draw upon prior memory to pattern match and then direct our muscles to make the appropriate movement. It is for this reason that plants don't have any need for brains. They get their food firmly rooted in one place and are effectively defenceless against any predators.

There is a type of sea mollusc, which has a tiny brain that helps it navigate the dark depths of the ocean to find a rock that it can call home. Once it finds the right rock, it attaches itself firmly to the rock and commits to spend the rest of its short life attached to it, thus eliminating any need for further locomotion. With this particular need gone, there is no need to still carry and maintain the energy-guzzling brain and hence the mollusc's body slowly digests the brain for energy. That image is worth keeping in mind for all the couch potatoes out there! If you are not moving, you are not using your brain for what it was evolved to do, and maybe, you don't need one either.

As humans, we have come full circle when it comes to movement. We have bodies that evolved for movement and brains that very delicately orchestrate this fine locomotion. Using this ability, we conquered continents, cleared large landmasses and established large, vibrant, thriving civilizations. But it always required work and movement. Until a few hundred years ago, nearly everyone had to work outdoors, just to make ends meet. Since most of our evolutionary history was spent hunting and gathering, that's what we did. We hunted and foraged, both of which require movement, until it was all outsourced, and now, we can get hunted (nay, farm-grown) meat, neatly packaged and delivered by BigBasket at our door step!

While all the energy saving devices have had a profound positive impact on our lives, they have also contributed to us becoming more and more sedentary. As the nature of work moved from agriculture to factory work to white collar office work, we have moved from using our whole bodies to only using our fingertips to type on a keyboard, and even that can be eliminated now, with voice diction software which I feel tempted to use even as I type this paragraph!

The irony of how far the whole approach towards movement and fitness has changed is illustrated by the history of how treadmills evolved. Devices similar to treadmills were first used by Romans to turn winches and lift heavy objects. These were adapted by a Victorian inventor named William Cubitt in 1818 to use in the punishment of prisoners, as a way to prevent idleness. For over 100 years, English convicts, including Oscar Wilde, spent hours a day trudging on treadmill-like devices with huge steps. Today we are happy to pay a monthly gym membership for the privilege (or punishment, depending on your perspective) of running on these treadmills, voluntarily!

Daniel Liberman is a palaeoanthropologist and Professor of Biological Sciences at Harvard University who has done pioneering and extensive research into how movement evolved, drawing on the fitness habits of communities who still follow the hunter–gatherer way of life. He has also studied our closest evolutionary cousins, chimpanzees, in the wild and written a fascinating book titled *Exercised: Why Something We Never Evolved to Do Is Healthy and Rewarding*. He reaches the conclusion that while surviving in the wild requires continuous movement to find food and mates as well as to avoid danger, we also simultaneously evolved to avoid movement whenever we could to conserve energy. It is not uncommon to see members of traditional tribal communities spend hours sitting and doing nothing after their daily chores are done. Similarly, chimps are inactive for as many as 8–10 hours a day, not counting sleep. But the difference is that for the few hours that they are active, they use their full body engaged in a whole range of movements. Humans in the wild and chimps don't exercise formally and are highly motivated to rest as much as they can to conserve precious energy. And yet, their lifestyles require many hours of labour-intensive work which keeps their bodies in top shape without any need for treadmills!

I grew up playing sports all my life. As soon as I came back from school, I would head to the playground and play all kinds of sports for as long as I could. I didn't know this back then but numerous studies have now confirmed the immense benefits of physical activity and being outdoors on brain and body health. As a result, I was always very lean and really enjoyed being physically active. In the first few years after I started working, my level of activity started dropping. I started to feel more fatigued and began to see the early signs of weight gain in all the wrong places. This was further compounded by my easy access to greasy fast food for every meal. Thankfully, around this time, my roommate got into bodybuilding and within six months, he was ripped. Inspired by his transformation, I joined him and thus started my tryst with learning everything I could about organized fitness.

I pursued a bodybuilding-style workout for a few years and eventually had plenty of muscles to show for it. But I also got bored just pumping iron in the gym, so I started experimenting with various other forms of exercise, starting with long distance running. I eventually worked my way up to half marathons (21 km) but never really progressed beyond this, as running non-stop for a couple of hours was triggering various repetitive stress injuries. From running, I moved to CrossFit, which is a high-intensity workout where you go all out for a few minutes, taking your heart rate very high, then taking a short break, followed by a repeat of the exercise. You feel quite winded after just a few rounds, but any type of HIIT work is amazing for heart health and is now highly recommended by fitness experts. I eventually tried every possible type of workout from combat sports to dance to yoga and Pilates, and I frankly enjoyed every form of being active, moving and being in tune with my body.

My quest to keep exploring different workout formats eventually landed me at CULT! When I was transitioning from Flipkart and contemplating my next venture CureFit, I used to go for long morning walks at a lake near my home. I used to see a new gym named CULT that had come up near the lake, which advertised Mixed Martial Arts (MMA) as its core focus area. I was intrigued and one day wandered in to inquire about how it worked. The person in charge asked me to enrol in a trial class, which was a set of drills inspired by rugby training. In one of the drills, I was paired with a giant of a man who must have weighed at least 100 kg, and the objective of the drill was to snatch the ball away. In the competitive spirit of not wanting to lose, I ended up wrestling on the ground with this large person on top of me and a rugby ball in between. After a minute of struggle, I felt something snap, and this turned out to be a hairline fracture in my rib. Fortunately, I eventually healed and went back to talk to Rishabh who had started CULT. In our conversations it became clear that if we simplified the format and expanded the range of offerings, we could make group workouts fun and accessible to everyone. That led to a long association with CULT, and we now run over 600 centres around the country and offer every possible type of workout in a safe, fun manner.

Fitness and movement form the backbone of any health regimen. In this chapter we will look at the science of fitness and various types of workouts that you can mix and match to design your own fitness journey.

On Sitting & Being Sedentary

In the recent past, warnings about the perils of sitting and being sedentary have reached a fever pitch. We are constantly bombarded by articles warning us that 'your chair is trying to kill you'[1] or that 'sitting is the new tobacco'[2]. There is no question that being sedentary all day is bad for us, as movement provides critical nourishment for both body and mind. But we should not blindly malign sitting either. Sitting is also an evolutionary artefact, and an energy-saving posture that our bodies have evolved. All animals in the wild sit for long stretches, especially if they are at the top of the food chain. Some years ago, I was on a safari in Kenya in a patch of the jungle filled with lions, but most of the lions we saw were just sitting around, looking regal as they lounged and took in the scenery around them. No one would accuse these lions of not being fit—something the hapless animals who are hunted down every few days would probably attest to. So, what does it mean? Should we sit or avoid sitting at all costs? Well, most things to do with health are nuanced and this is no exception.

We spend 8–10 per cent more calories when we are standing as compared to when we are sitting. That translates into thirty extra calories for four hours of standing per day or 10,000 calories over a year which equals more than a kilogram of weight loss! Conversely you can save this energy by sitting and give your body the rest it instinctively craves. The right balance is to split your waking hours in the ratio of 1:2, i.e., about five hours of activity, walking, standing or moving around and another ten hours of sitting in an easy, comfortable posture. Contrary to the myth of the 'savage athlete', most modern-day hunter–gatherers also sit for 8–10 hours a day. But what they don't do is sit on chairs with nice comfortable backrests. Backrests allow the back muscles to relax, and this has an adverse effect on overall body posture over a long period of time. Rural teenagers in Kenya, who rarely sit in chairs, have 21–41 per cent stronger backs than teenagers from the city, who spend most of their days in chairs. Studies also show that backrests demand less sustained muscular effort, so those of us who sit in chairs regularly have weak back muscles without endurance.

How you sit also matters. When anthropologists study various cultures around the globe, they find hundreds of different sitting postures; the most common ones requiring squatting or folding of the legs, both of which are great for leg stretches, as well as keeping the back upright and engaged.

There is no question that being sedentary all day is bad for you but sitting is an integral part of how we spend our days and it is not going away. After you get the requisite movement, you can be mindful about where and how you sit. Getting up frequently for short walks to keep your blood circulating better and experimenting with various sitting positions, including on chairs without backrests, might be a good idea to make sitting work for you.

* * *

THE SCIENCE OF MOVEMENT

The science of exercise has advanced by leaps and bounds in the recent past, revealing a wealth of information about how our bodies and minds respond to movement. When we exercise, we are engaging various muscle groups, joints and tendons of the body, moving them, stretching them, or placing them under a load of some kind. These movements impact almost every bodily function, from metabolism to the release of hormones, while also influencing the levels of neurotransmitters that impact the mind.

Exercise is based on the concept of placing controlled amounts of stress on the body, to which the body adapts. The best example of this is weight training. Lifting weight recruits a larger part of the muscle fibre than normal movement does, placing greater stress on the muscle. This leads to micro-tears in the muscle that are repaired after a workout, making it better adapted to the strain of the next workout. In most forms of exercise, this stress or load on the body is gradually increased to improve strength or endurance over time. The story of Milo of Croton beautifully illustrates this concept. As a young boy Milo began to carry a small calf on his shoulder everywhere he went, despite the ridicule of his peers. Gradually, however, the calf grew, and along with it, so did Milo's strength. As the story goes, Milo went on to enjoy a long and illustrious wrestling career, inspiring many and setting in stone the training principle of progressive overload.

Most forms of exercise take our heart rates up, and have a powerful effect on our cardiovascular health. In a fascinating study conducted way back in 1953, perhaps among the earliest looking at the relationship between heart health and physical activity, it was found that London bus drivers, who sat all day, had higher rates of heart disease than conductors on the same buses, who were constantly on their feet.[3] Similarly, it was found that postmen, whose jobs required physical activity, had a lower incidence of coronary heart disease than their colleagues sitting in government offices. I have recently adopted the habit of doing my meetings standing up as often as I can. While I did get some odd looks in the early days, it has now been accepted, and I occasionally see other folks stand up as well. Maybe standing meetings will be more of the norm in the near future.

While studies have shown a positive relationship between physical activity and longevity, the Copenhagen City Heart Study, conducted in 2015, found that there might be an optimal amount of cardio exercise for longevity.[4] They found that between one and two hours of jogging, two to three times per week, was associated with the lowest mortality. The researchers also discovered a U-shaped association between aerobic exercise and mortality. They found that light and moderate joggers had a lower mortality than sedentary individuals who did not exercise, while the mortality rate of 'strenuous' joggers was not statistically different from the sedentary non-joggers. In addition to longevity and heart health benefits, cardio training improves lipid profiles by lowering bad cholesterol and increasing good cholesterol. Studies have also found that cardio exercise can protect against brain atrophy and obesity. Ideally, 150–300 minutes of light to moderate intensity cardio workouts per week will yield the best benefits.

A quick aside here, to remember that achieving this general recommendation for exercise is not an excuse to become an 'active couch potato'. Exercising a few times a week cannot make up for an otherwise sedentary lifestyle. The best way to reduce the number of sedentary hours in our days is to simply move more often—whether this means walking to work, doing more household chores or even setting up standing meetings. The best way to reap the benefits of exercise is to become more active in your everyday life.

Exercise is a great way of increasing bone density, something that has been studied in the context of osteopenia and osteoporosis, conditions marked by the loss of bone density. In addition, menopausal women often develop osteoporosis, highlighting the importance of regular physical activity for middle-aged and older women. People with osteoporosis suffer frequent fractures, and exercise is of crucial importance, as it improves motor coordination which can prevent falls.[5] The two main categories of exercise that are best for bone health are weight-bearing cardio workouts like climbing stairs and jogging, and strength and resistance-based workouts, including lifting weights, or cycling and swimming.[6]

Apart from improved heart health, and stronger muscles and bones, exercise has some other wonderful benefits, including on the quality of sleep. Studies have found that moderate aerobic exercise improves sleep quality, by increasing time spent in slow wave or deep sleep. However, not only are the mechanisms of this unclear, but the effects of exercise on sleep also depend on intensity and timing. For example, late evening workouts could prevent good sleep because exercise raises core temperature which signals the body to wake up, while the release of various hormones could also make falling asleep harder.

We have somehow come to associate fitness and activity with young age and accepted that slowing down with age is just how things are meant to be. But a study of all indigenous societies around the world shows that that is not the case at all. In the Hadza hunter–gatherer communities of northern Tanzania, grandmothers forage more than mothers who are busy nursing and caring for their young children. Hadza grandfathers are as active as those of their sons' generation, hunting, collecting honey and walking long distances. Thus, they maintain higher levels of strength and fitness in old age than adults in industrialized societies. Similarly, in the animal kingdom, you don't see old and tired lions depending on their offspring to bring them food. The day the lion stops hunting is the day the lion dies.

The body of somebody who has never trained will peak in its twenties, and by age forty, everything will start to decline. By the age of fifty, muscles mass begins to diminish at the rate of 1–2 per cent per year, and 10 per cent or more per decade. However, our bodies continue to be adaptable even post mid-life. We can still build muscle, regaining the lost power and strength, but only if we take action—sooner rather than later. In fact, a 2007 study[7] identified almost 600 genes that play a role in skeletal muscles that change with age, many of which are specifically involved in metabolism and mitochondrial function. In the study, older male subjects underwent a six-month training regime that increased their strength by 50 per cent. At the end of the study, 170 of the identified genes had shifted into reverse, resembling those of much younger men. Another study[8] compared a group of older male subjects between the ages of sixty and seventy-one with healthy younger men. Both groups at the time were lifting weights. After twenty-two weeks of strength training, however, the older and younger subjects had comparable strength and muscle mass. In fact, some of the older subjects had better muscle thickness in their upper arms.

All of this goes to show that, no matter what your age, you can benefit from the effects of exercise. It's good for your heart and your bones, it keeps you feeling young and strong, and it might improve not just your health span but your lifespan too.

The Runner's High

I distinctly remember the incredible high I would feel after a run back in my running days. My entire head would be awash in feel-good emotions and I'd feel invincible. The sense of euphoria and oneness would make me want to come back and do it all again despite the gruelling ordeal that long-distance running is. This is what is known as the runner's high and the reason why long-distance running is so popular around the world. If you have ever experienced that rush of euphoria or sense of elation after a run or a particularly tough workout, you have witnessed the intricate link between the body and the mind in action.

In the last few decades, ultra running has gained a lot of popularity and has emerged as the bounce–back platform for various mid-life crises. Ultra running has shown that human bodies are immensely adaptable and, with the right kind of conditioning and training, we can get huge mileage out of our bodies. Ultra running not only helps with the physique and stamina, but can also boost confidence and self-esteem immensely. Additionally, most ultra running takes you away from the city into countryside, jungles and mountains, and just being in the presence of serene nature can melt away a lot of worries and anxieties.

Author Christopher McDougall's bestselling book *Born to Run* has done an incredible job of popularizing the sport of running and making the cutting-edge research into the sport available to large audiences. McDougall traces the running traditions of the Tarahumara—a lost tribe living in the Copper Canyons of Mexico. Far from urban life and industrialization, these people have incorporated running in some of their most sacred festivals and traditions. The Tarahumara run barefoot for very long distances without any apparent training. Since the publication of this book, other researchers have also studied the community and have argued that it is not that this tribe is born with running genes, but their active lifestyle in the rugged mountain terrain actively trains them—which is why it is no surprise that some of them can run long distances without the need to train like Western athletes. Most kids will agree! They run around all day without nary a worry about their running gait or landing skills.

One of the observations that experts have made is that the greatest marathoners in the world run like kindergartners. Ken

Mierke, an endurance coach, says that Kenyan runners run like children, pushing back as their feet land right under them. Unlike those of us who 'train' to run wearing expensive sneakers, they just continue to run the way they did growing up, and they do it barefoot.

Our bodies intuitively know how to run and this ability to run has conferred a huge evolutionary advantage. Incorporating some form of running in your routine is a great way to engage the body, get the heart rate up and even enjoy some meditative benefits as you keep one foot in front of another, letting your worries fade with every step.

FITNESS FOR BRAIN HEALTH

Working out might not just strengthen your muscles, but might also help your brain grow, quite literally. Exercise improves synaptic plasticity in the brain, both of which make you a better learner and improve your memory. This occurs through the stimulation of brain derived neurotrophic factor (BDNF) and other similar neurotrophins.

The cognitive and mood-boosting effects of exercise are caused by the increased levels of neurotransmitters post-workout. Dopamine is believed to be associated with motivation and reward in the context of exercise and might also improve cognition. Exercise also raises levels of serotonin, reducing feelings of anxiety and depression. Various other neurotransmitters are also involved in the delicate orchestration of brain function and mood, and exercise has a profound impact on these. However, studies have found differing results based on intensity, type and duration of exercise. For example, low intensity exercise might have the most beneficial effect on serotonin, thus improving mood and sense of wellbeing, while very intense exercise could have the opposite effect, causing stress.

Exercise is known to increase levels of cortisol, the stress hormone. Moderately elevated levels of cortisol are associated with improved learning and memory. An interesting observation that has been made is that those with higher levels of exercise-induced cortisol had the lowest levels of stress-induced hormone, which means they develop better resistance to unhealthy stress.[9] In fact, Andrew Huberman who is professor of neuroscience at Stanford, recommends a small burst of vigorous exercise just before a learning activity to boost learnability and retention.

Perhaps an area in which exercise has the most potential for impact is mental health. While research is ongoing, there is some evidence that more active people are less likely to be depressed than those who are more sedentary. In one 2007 study, 200 participants diagnosed with major depression were randomly assigned to one of four groups—one receiving supervised group training, one doing home-based exercise, one receiving antidepressant medication, and the last receiving a placebo pill.[10] After four months, the groups who exercised and who took antidepressants showed higher rates of remission, meaning they no longer fell into the category of people with major depressive disorder. The researcher followed up with participants a year later and found that those who had remained active showed lower levels of depression.

Exercise has also been found to be effective in the treatment and even prevention of anxiety and panic disorders, as well as post-traumatic stress disorder. Aerobic and strength workouts, as well as mind–body practices such as yoga, seem to improve, and alleviate symptoms related to depression and anxiety. The scope of the role of exercise in the management of mental health and wellbeing is vast, and only just being tapped.

HEALTH HACK #10: HaloSport

HaloSport claims that its headset can actually boost your neuroplasticity, or the ability of the brain to create new circuits to speed up learning. According to the brand, this nifty device can enhance skill learning, build strength and improve endurance, whether you're learning a new language, sport or instrument, or looking to improve your workouts.

Training Your Heart Out

On average, our hearts beat around seventy-two times per minute and do so for as long as we live. For an average lifespan that means about three billion beats in a lifetime. That is one hell of a strong organ—the one we literally can't live without. While we are all naturally endowed with this miracle of an organ, the wear and tear of our lifestyle catches up and most people's hearts start to struggle in later years, unless they do something about this. Being active and fit is just about the best thing you can do for your heart and you may reap decades of good health as a result.

Cardio or aerobic exercise—including brisk walking, jogging, running, cycling, swimming, dance workouts, circuit training and HIIT, as well as some forms of martial arts and most sports—takes the heart rate up, which does the body a world of good. When the heart rate goes up, the heart is forced to pump faster, thus strengthening its muscles. This may also clean up any debris in the arteries and expand them to make it harder for plaque to form. If we regularly train at high heart rates, this has the added benefit of reducing our resting heart rate (RHR) which is highly correlated with quality of sleep and the restfulness you feel after a good night's sleep. People who exercise regularly tend to have low resting heart rates and better aerobic capacity as their heart is able to pump more blood per contraction.

In addition to its direct impact on the cardiovascular system, exercise reduces risk factors that are associated with heart disease, such as obesity, hypertension and type 2 diabetes.[11] Exercise is also known to have anti-inflammatory effects, which, in turn, improves glucose and lipid metabolism.[12]

Heart rate zones for training are based on one's maximal heart rate—calculated by subtracting one's age from 220. The intensity of exercise is defined according to your maximum heart rate. The American College of Sports Medicine's recommendations for these zones are as follows[13]:

- Very light exercise: <57 per cent
- Light: 57–63 per cent
- Moderate: 64–76 per cent
- Vigorous: 77–95 per cent
- Near Maximal: >96 per cent

You can calculate your approximate maximum heart rate (MHR) by subtracting your age from 220. So, for someone who is forty years old, the MHR will be about 180.

If you're just starting out on your exercise or training regime, it might be best to start out easy, keeping yourself in the very light and light zones for a few weeks at least. If you're already training, the first zone is great for recovery days, while the light zone is the best way of increasing endurance over longer, sustained periods of time. It is also in the light zone that the body switches over to using fat as a fuel, so this is a good place to be if weight loss is your objective. Gradually, you can start pushing into the moderate zone, which is where you really start reaping the benefits of a cardiovascular workout. Staying in the moderate zone is a great way of improving your aerobic capacity and your stamina. In the vigorous zone, your body uses a combination of its aerobic and anaerobic capacity. Exercising in this zone pushes up the heart rate and really gets you sweating. And finally, the near maximal zone is what you reach when you push into high intensity interval training for short bursts of high energy exercise.

Another important concept in the context of cardiovascular fitness is heart rate variability (HRV), which refers to the variation in time between each heartbeat. This measure reflects the function of the autonomic nervous system–which includes the sympathetic nervous system that activates the fight-or-flight response as well as the parasympathetic nervous system with its relaxation response. The sympathetic nervous system speeds up heart rate while the parasympathetic system slows it down. When the body is stressed or on alert, HRV is low, while the variation between heart beats is higher when in a relaxed state. A higher HRV indicates a balanced autonomic nervous system and a body that is prepared to adapt to changes in the environment. Age, gender, lifestyle factors and fitness levels can influence HRV, with elite athletes having greater variability than non-athletes.

Many wearable devices now track heart rate variability, and those worn on the chest are believed to be more accurate than those worn on the wrist. It might be a good idea to monitor your HRV over a period, observing the effects of exercise or meditation on it over time. Apart from fitness and activities that combat stress like meditation, better nutrition, hydration and improved sleep can also improve HRV.

Building Muscles

In 1902, a ten-year-old named Angelo Siciliano landed in America from Italy. He spoke no English at the time, and moved into his uncle's Brooklyn home with his mother. Angelo fell ill often as a child, and regularly suffered beatings at the hands of his abusive uncle and school bullies. On one occasion, he wasn't able to protect a girl he was with at the beach and he was filled with shame. Impressed by the muscles of the Greek gods he saw at the Brooklyn Museum, Angelo aspired to become like them one day and started training rigorously.[14] Using weights, ropes and grips in his room, he spent some months training to little effect. He then had another moment of clarity while observing lions at the Bronx Zoo—wondering how they became strong without weights, he assumed they did so by 'pitting one muscle against the another'.

Angelo started experimenting with 'dynamic tension', what we now call isometric training, and he began to see incredible results. When a friend commented that he looked like the statue of Atlas atop the Atlas Hotel, he changed his name to Charles Atlas— the first muscleman of his era—and launched the physical culture movement. Charles Atlas became a model, started a mail-order course promising to help everyone achieve a muscular body, and inspired generations of fitness enthusiasts.

At first, people like Charles Atlas and many other muscle men who followed him were considered oddities, going around flexing their muscles for show or performing herculean feats for entertainment. But in the 1960s, bodybuilding started to get organized as a sport and finally burst into the mainstream. As people around the world came to realize the perils of sedentary lifestyles, they clamoured for nicer and more convenient places to workout, resulting in the massive proliferation of gyms around the world. Today, it's impossible to go to any city in the world and not find a large number of high-quality gyms.

In addition to losing weight, building muscle remains one of the most common goals shared by people starting out on their fitness journeys. Traditional gyms are still geared towards this, as evidenced by the equipment as well as the muscle-flexing you see in them. Fortunately, we now have much better science than Charles Atlas did back in his day, showing us how to build muscle for good long-term health and not just aesthetics.

When starting out, you can strengthen your muscles using your own body weight, doing variations of push-ups, squats, lunges, tricep dips, planks and more. Gradually and with the guidance of a trainer, you can start using weights such as dumbbells, kettlebells and medicine bells, as well as resistance bands.

Lifting weight recruits a larger part of the muscle fibre than normal movement does, placing greater stress on the muscle. This leads to micro-tears in the muscle that are repaired after a workout, making it better adapted to the strain of the next workout. This process of muscle growth is known as hypertrophy. If the micro-tears are too few because of a light workout, the body doesn't really adapt. At the same time, if too many micro-tears are caused, the body cannot fully repair the muscle, leading to a slowdown in muscle growth. Research has found that lifting heavy weights in sets of 4–6 reps resulted in the most increase in strength, or the most optimal micro-tearing leading to adaptation.[15] With weight training, short but intense workouts work best—one of those cases of 'less is more'.

In his research, Dr Duncan French, a performance specialist and Vice President of Performance at the UFC Performance Institute, found that six rounds of ten reps each at an intensity of 80 per cent, with two-minute breaks between rounds was the most beneficial protocol to create an anabolic environment in which muscle is built.[16] This protocol boosts testosterone and growth hormone and might be the ideal one to follow if muscle growth is your fitness goal. Dr French found that the more traditional German Volume Training plan of ten rounds of ten reps was not sustainable and might even be counterproductive.

There are many variations when it comes to weight training. Zero momentum reps (ZMR) refers to moving the weights very slowly so that you are not benefiting from the lifting momentum. There are many high repetition workouts where you take a low weight at 30–50 per cent of your one rep max (1RM—the heaviest weight you can lift with good form) and aim for as many reps as possible (AMRAP). These workouts are great for increasing heart rate, improving stamina and enhancing muscle tone.

Depending on what type of strength movement you engage in, you subject your muscles to different types of contractions. For example, in bicep curls, if you're curling the weight upward by flexing the elbow, the bicep muscle is generating force while shortening, known as **concentric** muscle action—how muscles move us. If you hold a weight steady without moving it up or down, the bicep muscles will try to shorten but won't change length, known as **isometric** action

By lowering weight very slowly, you engage an **eccentric** muscle action, firing the biceps as they lengthen. Concentric contractions are critical for movement but not as effective for building muscles. To get stronger, therefore, one incorporates eccentric and isometric movements. This means one should slow down the repetitions, hold the position for a few seconds at about 70 per cent of the contraction and bring down the weight as slowly as possible, and you will eventually have ripped muscles to show for the effort.

It has been shown that occasionally lifting very heavy weights can have a significant impact on the rate of muscle gains. Doing as many reps as possible at about 80 per cent of 1RM has been found to have a significant and lasting impact on muscle gain. But lifting heavy weights can be highly injury prone and it is best done with a trainer or workout partner.

In a typical muscle-building regimen, one may want to 'cut' (adjust the diet and add cardio to lose fat) or 'bulk' (adjust nutrition to maximize muscle gains and adding fat in the process). 'Maintaining' is the slow gaining of muscle while avoiding fat gain. Traditional strength programmes were based on periods of bulking and cutting, first consuming excess calories to bulk up, then going into a caloric deficit to lose fat. However, this is not a very sustainable programme for beginners and puts immense stress on the body. So, what's the deal: do we have to choose one or the other—muscle gains or fat loss?

Fortunately, newer schools of thought say you don't have to choose. 'Body recomposition' refers to gaining muscle and losing fat at the same time. These programmes are tailored to individuals and usually recommend a concurrent programme of strength and cardio training, combined with a balanced diet that is high in protein. Instead of focusing only on weight loss, which doesn't differentiate between the loss of fat and the loss of muscle, body recomposition training might require you to measure body fat and circumference of specific areas.

Studies have found that in people who have never trained with weights before, muscles respond dramatically and quickly to resistance training. Even without the excessive calorie consumption traditionally recommended for bulking, novices experience what is called 'newbie gains', putting on muscle mass while losing fat mass, all while in a calorie deficit. Those who have been doing resistance training for some years might need to experiment with their training and diet plan to figure out their own route to body recomposition.

In his very popular podcast on everything concerning neuroscience, fitness and health, Dr Andrew Huberman discusses harnessing the body's natural thermoregulation to boost performance. According to Dr Huberman, the skin tissue of our face, hands and feet release heat very quickly. So, during intense training, if you were to frequently splash your face with cold water or dip your palms in ice cold water for a few seconds, your body could lose built up heat and you would be able to exert a lot more in the next set. There are now even cooling mitts that you can wear in between sets to cool down your body faster. I have recently adopted the habit of immersing myself in an ice bath right after my workouts to accelerate post workout recovery.

When it comes to building muscle, recovery is almost as important as exercise and nutrition, because this is when your muscles repair themselves and get stronger. Ensuring that you get a good night's rest and treat muscle stiffness and soreness can help you see better gains from your workouts.

Sports for Fitness

When someone says they are really into sports, they usually mean they like to watch the sports on television, often well into the night, often with beer and pizza, thus using sports for the overall detriment of their health, the exact opposite of what it is supposed to do. It gets even worse with fantasy sport, betting real money and enjoying the thrill of gambling without lifting a muscle (if you don't count poking at your phone screen to make your fantasy team as effort). Don't get me wrong. I have nothing against watching sports. In fact, a lot of my happiest memories are of fanatically watching sports and following my favourite players and teams, often waking up very early to catch an important game. But your passion for sport should not end with television.

Most of us grow up playing games, and recreational sports are part of everyone's routines until daily adult life gets in the way and we resign ourselves to enjoy the thrill of playing only vicariously. But it doesn't have to be that way. Sports are one of the best ways to engage in physical and mental activities, not even counting the additional benefits of social interaction and being outdoors. If you could do only one thing for your fitness, playing a sport is just about the best thing you can do.

Play has been part of our evolutionary history as far as we can tell. Nearly every species of mammal demonstrates some form of play behaviour in childhood. You must have seen your dog chasing squirrels and fetching sticks, or monkeys swinging away to glory in the trees. Despite the energy expenditure involved in play-based activities, evolution has selected for this trait and for a good reason. Playing allows mammal infants to develop physical skills and capacities required for hunting or fighting as adults. It also teaches them to create cooperative bonds and defuse moments of tension.

If you played a sport as a kid, why not think about easing yourself back into it and making it a part of your lifestyle? Or you can learn a new sport altogether, keeping your brain sharp and agile by discovering and practicing new skills.

MOBILITY

Mobility is not a concept traditionally associated with fitness, unlike strength, endurance and speed. And yet, increasingly, mobility is being recognized as one of the pillars of fitness, no matter what one's goals are. Mobility of the body refers to the ability to perform functional movement patterns with full range of motion (ROM). In simpler words it is when a joint can move in all the ways it's supposed to be able to. It is the unrestricted movement of joints without being inhibited by the tendons, ligaments or muscles that surround them.

People often confuse mobility with flexibility. Flexibility refers to the ability of muscles to lengthen passively—think, for example, of stretching. Flexibility requires an external force in the form of a tool or another person to move connective tissue, and in that sense is a passive movement. In fact, flexibility might not be as important as it has historically been considered. The joint positions comprising what we call flexibility cannot be controlled by the nervous system and therefore don't improve movement and function in our bodies. When we talk about mobility, on the other hand, we're talking about a far more active capacity; one that involves the stability, coordination and control of the muscles that surround every joint as we perform a functional movement. Mobility comes under the direct control of the nervous system and can improve both flexibility and our ability to control different movement patterns. We have talked about how important movement is for the human body and having mobility means being able to move truly efficiently.

The importance of mobility comes to light in the context of the kinetic chain, a concept that describes the interrelated movements of joints with other joints, muscles, tendons and ligaments to create a movement pattern. Without mobility, this chain of movement breaks down. In order to 'compensate' for the mobility, another part of the body takes the hit, resulting in prolonged wear and tear, finally ending in injury. With better mobility, you don't just reduce your risk for injury, you also improve your strength, endurance, agility, and speed.

Many athletes suffer from a lack of mobility due to a lack of recovery from the intense work they put their body through during training and performance. In fact, immediately after a game, professional athletes and players can suffer a major loss of range of motion in the joints that were pummelled on the field or court. Thanks to the advances in sports science, more and more trainers and coaches are paying attention to exercises and workouts that address the kinetic chain and the mobility of joints.

According to the joint-by-joint approach conceptualized by strength and conditioning coach Michael Boyle and explained by Gray Cook in his book *Movement*, the body is envisioned as a systematically stacked structure of joints. Each joint or system of joints has a specific function and is prone to specific kinds of dysfunction, and thus each must be trained in a certain way. And this is what tends to go wrong in traditional training programmes. According to this theory, the foot requires stability, the ankle requires mobility, the knee requires stability, the hips need mobility and so on, all along the kinetic chain. So, for example, a lack of ankle mobility will cause the knee—a stable joint—to move or cave in, leading to injury or inefficient movement. Approaching your training through the lens of the joint-by-joint approach can truly improve quality of movement.

FIND YOUR FORMAT

Now that we are armed with a basic understanding of what exercise can do for us, we get to the hard part—how to choose the right format for your health goals. The twenty-first century has seen an explosion in the world of fitness, with more and more choices when it comes to how, when and where we want to workout. With an array of formats to pick from, and technology becoming a powerful tool, the sky really does seem like the limit. For someone starting on their fitness journey or looking for a change in routine, this can be overwhelming.

For those who haven't exercised for a long period or anyone struggling with health issues of any kind, don't underestimate the power of a walk. While walking is a dynamic activity that engages almost all the muscle groups in a rhythmic movement, and which, according to some estimates, requires the use of over half the body's muscle mass, it is incredibly easy to incorporate it in everyday life.[17] With the rise of wearable devices, the 10,000-steps-a-day movement has sparked a revolution of sorts, validating the age-old activity of walking. I have observed that getting 10,000 steps a day is sufficient cardiovascular exercise for most people. I also find, personally, that if I have had a vigorous workout on a particular day, I feel winded and exhausted if I attempt to get 10,000 steps. That's why I'd recommend doing 10,000 steps on days that it is your only exercise, but fewer on days that you're hitting the gym.

Swimming is a form of very low impact cardio and also great for recovery from injury, while dance workouts can be immensely fun and a great way to sweat while listening to music and even making friends. Swimming is great for people who regularly travel as most hotels have a swimming pool, so this workout travels easily on holidays. After all, who doesn't like chilling in a pool or fancy an ocean swim during their downtime. Running is equally accessible and doesn't need anything to begin with. You can run anytime, anywhere as long as you have a pair of comfortable shoes—for proponents of barefoot running, even those are optional! Another benefit of running is that you can start as slow as you want. I know people who started with just a brisk walk or slow motion jogging after decades of doing nothing and then gradually paced up over months to be able to do a 10-kilometre run or even a full marathon. The journey of transformation is simply breath-taking, especially when considering the impact on mood and self-esteem.

When it comes to choosing what kind of workout is best for you, there is really no right answer. Today we have numerous fun and easily accessible methods available to engage and train any part of the body in a safe and effective manner. The starting point for most beginners is some form of strength training. The easiest way to start weight training is to use your body weight. When you perform a squat or a push-up, for example, you are lifting your body with the strength of your leg muscles or chest muscles. Another safe way to start weight training is to use machines that allow you to progressively load weights with a controlled range of motion, thus reducing the chances of injury. Most advanced forms of weight training use free weights, such as dumbbells, barbells or kettlebells. In addition to an optimal level of training, the body also needs adequate rest and good nutrition for healthy muscle growth.

What works best greatly varies from person to person. I might benefit most from strength training workouts, while someone else might thrive on a routine of long-distance runs. Not only do different exercise regimens suit different people and goals, but some people might find that changing up their routines every now and then is most effective. So, remember, start slow, and get some advice from an expert on form as well as warming up and cooling down (which can help prevent injury and chronic pain). If you're serious about your training, you could also think about combining your running regime with yoga and some strength training to take care of your muscles, joints, flexibility and strength. Armed with just the basics and a supportive, comfortable pair of shoes, you can begin your own running journey.

Some forms of fitness take things back to the basics, like functional training which is designed to improve function in your everyday movements, rather than just focusing on building muscle or getting lean.[18] Instead of training isolated muscles, you train with compound movements that imitate the movement patterns of daily living. If you think about it, it's unlikely that you will ever need to move your arm in real life the way you do for a bicep curl at the gym. However, you might squat down to pick something up, reach up above you for something else, or hinge slightly at the hips to lift up a heavy suitcase.

HOW LONG DOES FITNESS LAST WITHOUT EXERCISE?

A team of researchers in 2018 conducted a randomized control trial to understand the physiological effects of taking a break from a regular fitness regimen. It turns out, the benefits of exercise disappear within about a month of stopping your usual workout routine! In the study, all participants joined a thirteen-week personalized training programme, on completion of which they were randomly assigned either to a group that continued the programme for four weeks or to one that stopped training and did not perform any planned exercise for four weeks. After a month without exercise, and despite the gains they had made during the thirteen-week regimen, the researchers found a loss of training adaptations in members of the 'detrain' group. The benefits they had accrued with regards to blood pressure, high-density lipoproteins and triglycerides were completely lost in the four weeks with no workouts.[56]

Recent research has proven that incorporating high intensity interval training (HIIT) into your workout can maximize health and fitness benefits. The single most powerful health effect of HIIT is on cardiorespiratory health, specifically by improving VO2 max (which is the maximum amount of oxygen the body can use during exercise)—and improved VO2 max has a positive effect on overall health. HIIT is known to burn calories more effectively than continuous-pace workouts. For an even more time-saving workout, there is reduced exertion high intensity training or REHIT which includes fewer and shorter bouts of high-intensity exercises. A REHIT workout is usually a ten-minute session—including warm up and cool down—taking the form of two to three bouts of twenty-second cycle sprints. While research into REHIT is still in early stages, initial studies suggest that these super quick workouts can deliver cardiorespiratory benefits, even in the span of a few weeks and even in the case of individuals with sedentary lifestyles.[19]

Most cultures of the world have deeply thought about health, rigorously experimented and codified best practices into various fitness regimens, often combining physical, mental and even spiritual aspects into one comprehensive lifestyle. Growing up in Haridwar, I was exposed to yoga at a very young age but the idea of contorting my body into weird shapes didn't make much sense to me back then. It is only now that I understand the deep logic behind combining breath work with the body's strength and balance, that I have made yoga an integral part of my fitness regimen.

The field of yoga has been the site of fascinating research recently. In several studies, yoga was found to alleviate the symptoms of chronic pain, as well as to reduce inflammation, which is one of the causes of several chronic ailments. In addition, research has found that yoga has positive effects on heart health, hypertension and diabetes. [20] Tai Chi, an ancient martial art described as 'poetry in motion', can improve bone health, reduce blood pressure and improve heart health even in those with prior cardiovascular conditions.[21] Particularly in older adults, there is evidence that this practice improves balance and reduces risk of falls, while also having a positive effect on chronic illnesses like diabetes and osteoarthritis. If ancient martial arts are your thing, there are several more to choose from, including kalaripayattu and qi-gong.

Combat training, including practices like muay Thai, boxing and Brazilian jiu jitsu, are known not only to challenge the body's physical prowess but also to sharpen the focus of the mind. When choosing your fitness regime, don't forget to look at more traditional forms of sports such as tennis or cricket, which are great opportunities for full-body training while offering opportunities for social connection. If you love adventure and the outdoors, trekking, climbing and even surfing are excellent ways of engaging both body and mind for fitness.

Another form of training, Pilates, has gained popularity in recent years. Pilates was created by Joseph Pilates almost 100 years ago combining his knowledge of gymnastics with strength training. He devised speciality equipment that helps with core strengthening, stretching and engaging mind and breath to control the movements. Pilates has been quite popular among dancers and athletes as it seems to strengthen you from deep within, much like yoga. I have started learning Pilates recently and I can see it being part of my workout routine for a long time to come.

Being able to measure and track your fitness will help you make more informed decisions about your workouts and better progress overall. Some trainers suggest keeping a fitness journal, keeping track of how much you're lifting, how long you're maintaining high performance, your weight or circumference, your energy levels and your rest days. Some people even recommend taking photographs so you can see how your body transforms—as a visual motivator to stay on track.

PERIODIZATION

It's clear that for any high performance, a plan for training and recovery can keep you in the best form to achieve everything you set out to. Elite performers subject their bodies and minds to the most intense challenges, and this can sometimes make them more vulnerable in some ways. Periodization is considered one of the most effective strategies to develop an athlete's peak performance, focusing on a very specific schedule, based on performance or competition dates, to reduce risk for injury and improve overall fitness. This plan includes details on when to switch from general to sports-specific training, how to incorporate enough time for recovery to prevent fatigue, and how to manage volume loads to achieve the desired results. Periodization is a long-term, progressive approach to training, usually implemented alongside detailed nutrition plans and recovery schedules, to optimize performance.

Research has found that even elite athletes cannot sustain their peak performance for more than two or three weeks at a stretch. Given this, and the fact that competition dates determine when they need to be at their best, periodization is the ideal strategy to maximize performance. In general, periodization is divided into macrocycles (a season of training and competition), mesocycles (a training block within a season) and microcycles (a week of training).

In most training schedules based on periodization, there is an inverse relationship between volume and intensity. This means that as the competition nears, training intensity increases, while training volume decreases—shifting from an extensive to intensive workload. Periodization is also usually defined by a progression from general physical training to more sport-specific and technique training as the competition approaches. Depending on the schedule of training, which happens in cyclic periods, there is usually a fixed period of recovery, to prevent the onset of fatigue and to allow for adaptation to occur.

The Six-Pack & Beach Body

When it comes to working out, it's natural that many people have aesthetic objectives and are exercising in the hope of looking a certain way. The problem is that we have been exposed to entirely unrealistic physiques thanks to the internet, powerful marketing strategies and, of course, social media. Two of the most enduring ideas when it comes to fitness and aesthetics are the six-pack and the beach body.

Having enough definition for that elusive six-pack requires less than 10 per cent body fat, which is considered extremely unhealthy, especially for women.[22] In some cases, the side effects include severe hormonal changes and anxiety. Achieving the six-pack becomes an unhealthy obsession for many and might mean being on what is effectively a starvation diet. In addition, most people assume that certain classic movements like crunches and sit ups will work the core and lead to those chiselled abs, but the truth is that the core is a more complex group of muscles, and its health is not dependent on that much definition.

The beach body craze is another narrowly defined goal that is purely aesthetic, and often simply a short-term one. People often go on crash diets in the month before a holiday, only to start eating junk again when they return or even while on that holiday with sumptuous brunch buffets, endless happy hours and the irresistible allure of margaritas on the beach! There's nothing wrong with wanting to look 'fabulous' on your beach vacation, but the fact is, the unreasonable obsession with these short-term aesthetic driven goals may cause more harm than good. Do you want to be fit, healthy and live a better quality life, or do you just want to look great in those Instagram selfies? If you adopt fitness as a long-term lifestyle, you will get healthier in the long run and the aesthetic goals will just happen as a by-product. There is no short cut here. Fitness is something that ought to be part of your lifestyle, just like brushing your teeth or watching a movie is. If you are generally fit and know your way around the gym, there is no harm in putting in some extra effort before your holiday or a big event to shed a few pounds or sharpen your muscle tone. It feels great to look good, provided you do it the right way.

Whatever your health goals might be, I hope that this book will give you some food for thought in terms of how holistic wellbeing can truly transform the health of your body and your mind. When you change your habits and your lifestyle for better health, you will reap benefits that go far beyond looking good in a bathing suit or having a chiselled midriff. And once you experience that level of health, you'll never look back.

NEXT LEVEL STIMULATION: EMS

Electro muscle stimulation, known as EMS, is a type of training that uses a wearable device which delivers electrical impulses to directly stimulate the motor neurons, eliciting a muscle contraction. The tiny electrodes in the EMS device boost oxygen and blood flow to the muscle, causing a deep contraction, known as the 'squeeze', even during lower intensity workouts. EMS works by mimicking the action potential of the central nervous system—when a neuron is fired, sending electrical impulses along its axon to, in this case, contract the muscle. In comparison to traditional training methods, EMS targets all the body's large muscle groups and can reach even deeper lying muscle tissues, that are usually not easy to engage. While EMS is not a replacement for regular fitness—and probably doesn't lead to weight loss, as is often advertised—it can help boost the gains of strength training, even for those recovering from injury or older individuals.

HEALTH & EXTREME ATHLETES

David Goggins is an ex-US Navy SEAL, one of the world's most admired endurance athletes and the author of the book, *Can't Hurt Me*. But he wasn't always as strong and fit as he is now. In fact, as a young man, he was overweight, living on junk food and struggling to make ends meet, working as an exterminator. Goggins had a few years of military experience in the US Air Force, but it was a TV show about Navy SEALs that inspired him to enlist again and changed his life forever. Goggins realized that he would have to lose 45 kg in order to meet the basic fitness requirements and undergo some of the most famously gruelling training. The most challenging aspect of the programme is known as Hell Week, a whopping 130 hours of non-stop training on restricted food and sleep. Goggins had to participate in three Hell Weeks in a single year, dropping out of two because of illness and injury. But he was laser-focused, almost obsessed, and completed Hell Week on his third try, before going on to complete another!

The transformation—both physical and mental—inspired Goggins to keep going. After two decades of serving as a SEAL, he began to take part in some of the most challenging ultra-events to honour his fellow SEALs who had tragically lost their lives. In 2006, he competed in Badwater, described as 'the world's toughest foot race', a 136 mile course in the Death Valley of California where the soaring temperatures have been known to melt the soles of shoes right off. He went on to compete in the Ultraman World Championship on the Big Island of Hawaii—a three-day stage race comprising a 6.2 mile swim, a 260 mile cycle ride, and a 52.4 mile run, all in all more than twice the distance of an Ironman event. Despite never having competed in a triathlon event, Goggins finished second. The Ultraman event has no prize money, no media coverage and requires participants to support themselves with their own crews, making it more of a deeply personal physical challenge and spiritual quest than a public display of strength. Goggins' mental and physical determination in the face of the most extraordinary challenges show us the potential of the human mind and body in the face of the seemingly impossible.

The human body is often likened to the body of a car or some other piece of complex machinery, which can be fine-tuned to reach specific speeds or achieve certain feats. Yet, a car has very clear limits, and when pushed beyond these, will break down. Humans, however, seem to be constantly pushing against their limits. They appear to draw on some deep inner strength just at the point one would expect them to collapse. And this is what makes the field of human endurance so fascinating. There are many things that go into great performance—deliberate practice, mindset, willpower, working with a coach, optimizing the learning process and more. However, the element that is crucial for every elite athlete, and may actually be the foundation for high performance, is good health.

Performance requires not only showing up for training day after day, but also training just beyond one's comfort zone— something best done under the watchful eye of an expert coach who knows how much to push and when to stop. It can be painful, but the body will keep adapting to the new workload by building the infrastructure it needs.

Rich Roll is a world-famous ultra-marathon runner whose book, *Finding Ultra,* is a bestseller about the mindset and training for endurance sports. Rick argues that doing ultra distance running is as much about finding who you are as it is about the incredible endurance that is required for crazy distances such as 100 miles or more. While any ultra distance runner needs to get all the basics of strength, conditioning, and diet right, the mental side of training is equally important. If one plays the long-term game and keeps getting incrementally better every week, you will be shocked to find out what your body can do. Most ultra-marathoners start in their middle years, often spurred into action by decades of sedentary lifestyle, and gradually go on to running unimaginable distances. Sure, they end up punishing their bodies to the brink but they also get to know what they are made out of and usually see the positive impact of endurance training on every other aspect of their life as well.

But every time you push yourself, you risk injury and extreme fatigue. The reason something is beyond your comfort zone is that you don't yet have the trained capability to do what you are trying to and hence the struggle and exertion. If you end up pushing a bit beyond what your body can tolerate, you can end up with an injury which will offset your plans by weeks or months. This is where a good warm-up routine, regular mobility, stretching exercises and the guidance of a coach can be immensely helpful. You are looking for that Goldilocks zone which is just right, to train hard and effectively, without causing serious injury.

By training at extreme levels, you cause enormous stress to your body and mind, and it is important that you take recovery as seriously as training. The more you invest in recovery, the better prepared you'll be when you show up for your next training session, fresh and raring to push yourself again and again.

The Cost of Performance Training

While we all applaud the intensity and commitment with which elite athletes train, what we see as spectators is just a tiny sliver of long and often arduous journeys—not just physical, but mental and emotional as well. There is a very fine line between safe and unsafe training, and even a small misstep can put an athlete in serious danger. Fortunately, athletes now have both robust science and expert coaches on their side to ensure they are both safe and successful in their regimen and performance.

Training for performance involves the overload principle, which means constantly pushing the body just slightly beyond its current capacity. This very gradual increase in difficulty or load is considered a safe overload, and, done day in and day out, will add up to big changes and achievements. However, pushing too fast without proper preparation and planning can lead to injury, chronic conditions and overtraining as well. Overtraining is not just the result of too many sessions of intensive physical or mental practice, but of a poorly planned training schedule that does not sufficiently prioritize rest and recovery. Overtraining is associated with a sudden rise in inflammation as well as the rapid onset of fatigue, a condition in which athletes find it hard to keep up with their own speed and intensity. Studies have found that just four weeks of overtraining can cause damage to the body's cells, with disastrous consequences including oxidative damage and telomere shortening.

If you train too much, too hard and don't get enough rest, you could end up with overtraining syndrome (OTS). With OTS comes chronic fatigue, poor performance, frequent bouts of cold and flu, as well as mood swings and overall ill health. OTS is essentially a form of burnout, and its effects can last up to years. It has profound negative impacts on the quality of sleep as well as the immune system.

I have had numerous injuries over the years due to overtraining, pushing a particular movement beyond the breaking point or training with errors in form. These injuries have derailed my workout regimen by weeks and severely impacted my mood— and I can tell you, it's just not worth it.

What all of this means is that you cannot think about fitness without also thinking about recovery. After all, the gains from training are banked during the rest and recovery period. During training, you are just loading your muscles and causing small micro-tears or taking the muscle to near fatigue. It is only when you are resting that the body gets to do its repair work, improving the strength of the parts involved and slightly boosting performance after every cycle. In the next section, we'll take a deeper dive into the science of recovery and the protocols that you can incorporate in your life.

THE SCIENCE OF RECOVERY

Before we delve deeper into the subject of recovery, let's take a moment to understand what exactly goes on in the body that makes recovery a necessity. You might have heard about the concept of homeostasis—the constancy of our body's internal environment in spite of a changing external environment. The relatively constant temperature that our body maintains is one example of homeostasis. Stressors of various kinds tend to disrupt this internal balance of the body, ranging from illness, which is a bad kind of stress, to exercise, which we know can be a good form of stress. These stressors can interfere with the functioning of various physiological systems. Recovery is the process of returning the body to a state of homeostasis. When we follow the doctor's orders after a bout of illness, we are attempting to do just this. In this chapter, however, we will focus on a slightly different kind of recovery—recovering from workouts that take a toll on our bodies and minds.

In her book *Good to Go: What the Athlete in All of Us Can Learn from the Strange Science of Recovery*, science journalist Christine Aschwanden talks about how she observed the evolution of the idea of recovery. Recovery went from being a noun—a word almost synonymous with rest, relaxation and doing nothing—to being a verb. Suddenly everyone is 'doing' recovery. And while this is a great thing—that recovery is getting almost as much attention as training itself—it seems to come with a significant amount of stress and anxiety. We're all worried about whether we're recovering right, or enough, or in the optimum ways, and of course we are bombarded with often conflicting information. We are also bombarded with advertisements for every imaginable recovery device, supplement and tool out there! Despite this barrage of pseudoscience and marketing, there is also a lot of cutting-edge research on recovery. But what we need to do is learn to listen to our bodies better, getting back in tune with our own physiology, to understand when we need a time out or when we're ready to push harder. Most importantly, our recovery should bring us a deep sense of relaxation rather than more stress.

While we live in a time of incredibly advanced technology and have health metrics literally at our fingertips, some research suggests that there is something that is an even better measure of our recovery than objective statistics like heart rate or lactate levels—our mood. In addition to using the technology available to us to gauge how we feel, we should also be asking ourselves that question, and then using our own mood awareness to gauge what our recovery levels are. For example, if you're constantly irritable, grumpy or stressed, perhaps you haven't slept enough or taken enough of a break, whether from training or the stress of your workdays. If you are feeling fresh and energized, it's likely you are well rested and ready to take on some physical and mental work! For true recovery, the first and most important element is getting sufficient good-quality sleep. We will dive deeper into the science and best practices for sleep in the next chapter.

Beyond mood, there are also a few other useful measures of recovery. For the days that you aren't sure about whether your body has recovered enough to train again, Dr Andrew Huberman, a neuroscientist and a professor at Stanford, has some fantastic tips. To assess what he refers to as 'systemic recovery'[23], he recommends two simple tests you can conduct yourself, as soon as you wake up in the morning.

The first is a test of grip strength, in which you see if you are able form a tight fist or squeeze down hard on an object. This is a great indicator of your recovery because it reflects the control of the upper motor neurons over the lower motor neurons (responsible for motor movement) and whether the pathways from nerves to muscles have recovered from rewiring themselves. If you find yourself unable to form a tight grip or if you notice the strength weakening over a period, you might need to take a day or two off from your training regimen. One of the things I do before my training is grab the weighing scale in my hand and press it between my thumb and fingers as hard as I can and notice the scale. Whenever I am able to get past 20 kg, I know I am feeling well-recovered.

The second test is known as a CO_2 tolerance test, also done first thing in the morning. While lying down or sitting comfortably, take four deep breaths, inhaling through the nose and exhaling through the mouth. On the fifth breath, inhale as deeply as possible, expanding your diaphragm, and then start the timer as you exhale as slowly as possible through the mouth (tip: make a small 'o' with your lips as you would while drinking through a straw). You stop the timer when you cannot exhale anymore, measuring CO_2 discard rate or blow-off time. If you reach this point within twenty-five seconds or less, you might not have fully recovered from your last workout or the stress of everyday living. If you record a time of thirty to sixty seconds, you're in the clear to work out, and if you time is over sixty seconds, then you are well recovered and ready to do more physical work. For both these tests, it's a good idea to do them over the period of a few days and keep a record in a journal.

The CO_2 tolerance test is a test of your ability to engage the parasympathetic arm of the autonomic nervous system, putting a break on your stress. It turns out that this ability to tap into this part of the nervous system is a great tool for recovery—not surprising because we know that the parasympathetic nervous system initiates the relaxation response.

Dr Huberman recommends a few other methods of disengaging at the end of a training session and engaging the parasympathetic nervous system. Non-sleep deep rest is a state of deep relaxation also known as shallow sleep, in which one slows down the brain and the body while remaining in a conscious but not alert state. This is basically what is done in the practice of Yoga Nidra, and there are now studies that prove its powerful effects on the brain and body. Another tool that Dr Huberman recommends is doing ten physiological sighs—two inhales through the nose followed by a slow exhale—at the end of a training session.

Some amount of soreness about 12–24 hours after a workout is normal and termed delayed onset muscle fatigue or DOMS. Symptoms of DOMS include tender muscles, swelling, reduced range of motion in the muscles and joints you worked out and muscle fatigue. The body responds to the micro-tears in your muscles by increasing inflammation in those areas, which is believed to cause DOMS. However, if you find that your soreness lasts longer or feels more acute, it's best to consult a doctor.

As you figure out the best recovery practices and techniques for yourself, the only advice I have is to listen to your body, get enough sleep and keep a sceptical eye out for anything that sounds like it's promising magical recovery!

HEALTH HACK #11: Sauna

Saunas are believed to have originated around 2,000 BC in northern Europe, where they provided warmth and sterilized cave dwellings where important events took place. Saunas have several health benefits, including recovery, pain relief and improved blood circulation in the body.

PRACTICING RECOVERY

The human body is pretty amazing and is able to repair itself from wear and tear in almost magical ways, from the way a cut scabs over until it seems as though the wound never existed, to the way your stomach heals itself from an infection without medication. However, as we age, and as we engage in activities that go beyond natural wear-and-tear, we need to aid and even boost recovery to ensure we stay at the top of our games. A marathon, for example, is not a normal amount of exertion for the body. Pushing ourselves constantly, without giving our self-repair mechanisms time to kick in, could lead to serious and long-term health effects, including on our immune and nervous systems. Recovery, therefore, is more than protecting yourself from aches, pains and injury. It is also about shoring up every aspect of health through a rigorous regime.

Lately, the science of recovery has received a great deal of attention, and many health hacks focus on recovering, not only from the strenuous workouts we often subject ourselves to, but also from the wear and tear of everyday life. We face multiple stressors, from our lifestyles and environment, to work pressures and lack of sleep, each of which takes its toll on the body and mind. For good long-term health, recovery is as important as, or even more important than, an active lifestyle. Without a recovery plan, intense activity will run you down, leaving you exhausted and exposed, susceptible to reduced immunity and faster ageing.

Modern athletes take their recovery very seriously, whether it involves regular massages and travelling physiotherapists, or ice baths and red light therapy. For some, like Roger Federer and Tom Brady, their recovery happens during the ten to twelve hours a night they sleep, to let their bodies heal from the beating it takes on the court and field.

Pushing our minds and bodies out of their comfort zones through intense periods of training results in the release of the hormone cortisol. Cortisol boosts performance in the moment but also initiates the stress response, with a host of physiological effects. When we workout, our muscles accumulate micro-tears that need to be repaired for the muscle to grow. Repeated movements, like those performed at the gym, lead to the tightening of muscles that eventually knot together and form a lump. This can cause pain and affect performance and range of motion. Beyond physical activity, even our posture as we sit at our desks or the quality of the air we breathe on our commute can deplete our body's resources.

Recovery requires acknowledging the natural stressors in our lives and proactively working to stem their effects. The good news is that we now have all kinds of tools at our disposal. From ancient recovery techniques to modern gadgets, we have a plethora of options to pick from. Even though sleep and meditation remain the most potent recovery tools, there are many others that are well suited to specific stressors or matched to specific health goals. Here are a few for you to choose from.

Recovery techniques vary from the more basic at-home foam rollers and heat packs, to ancient methods now backed by science such as saunas and steam baths. And then there is the next level of recovery, with devices that often look like they came out of a futuristic, sci-fi graphic novel. Research into many of these is still in early stages, and there are several tech companies working on exciting new products, so this is a fascinating area to follow, and I, for one, am staying tuned.

After an intense workout, one of the simplest things to do is perform a few minutes of soft tissue mobilization using a foam roller or similar device. You can spend 10–20 seconds on each muscle region and more time on particularly tender spots. Another great tip is to roll a tennis ball beneath your feet—this releases tension and improves lower body range of motion. Stretching is another important part of post-workout recovery and doesn't require any equipment. Stretching lengthens muscles that might shorten and tighten during exercise. It's best to hold each stretch for about thirty seconds, and to avoid stretching regions that are especially painful in case of injury.

Compression therapy might be the next big thing in the prevention of DOMS. Wearing a garment that applies compression to specific body parts in a balanced and accurate manner can boost blood flow, which in turn increases the oxygen available to muscles. This leads not only to better performance, but allows muscles to sustain higher levels of performance for longer periods while speeding up muscle repair.

Saunas are enclosed rooms with high temperatures and low humidity, usually attached to spas, hotels or gyms, though they have been used by humans for thousands of years. They are excellent, not just for post-workout recovery to relax sore muscles and relieve tension, but also for general well-being, boosting cardiovascular health and immunity. Steam baths, that have high humidity levels and slightly lower temperatures compared to saunas, have similar benefits, while also being great for skin health.

Ice baths have been a favourite of elite athletes for some time now, but more and more people are recognizing their value. They have gone from simple tubs filled with ice, to more high-tech equipment that people can use at home and even travel with. Studies on athletes—including martial arts competitors and rugby players—have found that ice baths reduce the intensity of DOMS and muscle fatigue, thus speeding up recovery. While research is ongoing, an ice bath does bring immediate relief, boosts relaxation and can improve sleep. Taking it a notch up is cryotherapy, usually administered in a professional setting. The mechanism at work is the same that ice baths use—cold exposure leads to vasoconstriction or constriction of blood vessels, lowering the inflammatory response.

Massages are part of many ancient healing traditions, and while the jury is still out on their effectiveness, there is no doubt that they boost relaxation and relieve stress. When muscle tension and knots become chronic, physical therapists might recommend dry needling, in which a fine needle is inserted deep into the belly of a muscle to break the scar tissue and separate the fibres that might have fused to create that knot.

In addition to these, there are some very cool high-tech devices that can be used at home. You can choose from hand-held percussive 'guns' that can be linked to apps on your phone, electric muscle stimulators that boost recovery from injury and compression boots. There are even specially designed mattresses to transform your recovery journey. For days you don't have time to get in a workout or if you're feeling fatigued or unwell, you can try using a neuromuscular stimulation device (NMES) which mimics the muscular contractions of exercise. This can boost lymphatic drainage of cellular waste that builds up with intense exercise and speed up blood flow for healing.

If the pain or soreness after a workout feels more than usual, and you suspect you have an injury, it's best to check with your doctor or physiotherapist before picking a recovery method most suitable to your injury or ailment. It is sometimes apt to think of the body as a machine. Just as a machine requires periodic maintenance, our bodies, which undergo a lot of regular wear and tear, do too. As we go about our day-to-day activities or workouts, we accumulate damage and stress which add up. Recovery plays a crucial role in the long-term health of the body and mind, whatever form it may take.

HEALTH HACK #12: Get Some Sun

The best way to get some sunlight is to spend between five and thirty minutes outdoors in the morning sun. You could combine this with your exercise or a quiet walk in nature which has its own benefits, ensuring that your face, arms, legs and back (if possible) are exposed to the sun.

BIOMECHANICS

Our bodies are basically biomechanical machines that can pull off many interesting feats such as jumping on the two hind limbs and landing perfectly, curving and twisting the entire arm and torso and unleashing it at a fierce speed to throw a curveball at 100 mph or balancing in the tree pose on one limb for minutes at a time. All of these are the result of well-coordinated push and pull forces between various muscles, tendons and ligaments. Each movement requires a kinematic sequence in which a whole host of muscles fire in a particular chain causing a variety of pull–push motions and creating the right kind of tension against the muscular structure to affect the motion.

Our bodies have evolved to be able to execute these motions in a particular manner, honed by eons of evolution to result in this highly fine-tuned biomechanical apparatus that is breath-taking in its sophistication. But the same apparatus is also highly adaptable, responding beautifully to how it is used, and this is where things can go wrong. For example, in overhead movements, it is more efficient to use the upper back muscles, but for some reason, you start using more of your shoulder. The more you do it, the more the body gets trained to use the shoulder muscles where the back is supposed to be used. The back muscles have a lot more shock absorbers compared to the shoulders, which have some very tight and small muscles attached to the joint, which come under enormous strain. Incorrect biomechanical movements of this kind can lead to continuous wear and tear, which can eventually cause a serious injury, which is exactly what happened to my left shoulder.

Even though I have very strongly recommended fitness as a way of life, it is equally important to learn to do every movement well. There are people who land on their heels while running, or who don't engage the glute muscles while deadlifting, and so on which can lead to injury in the long run. In fact, the science of sports medicine is so advanced now that one can even predict future injuries based on a simple analysis of how biomechanics is being deployed today. The good news is that, by working with a good sports science physio or trainer, you can correct your posture and prevent yourself from getting a serious injury in the future.

Repetitive Stress Injuries

Certain kinds of training in some sports involve repeated actions and overuse that affect tendons, ligaments or muscles, most often in the hands or arms, causing repetitive stress injuries or RSIs. Tennis elbow and golf elbow are classic examples of these RSIs and are most often caused by a lack of sufficient rest and recovery after a period of intense training. As a result, the body doesn't have enough time to repair the micro-tears in the part being repeatedly worked. There was a period in my life where I would practice my golf swing for hours on the driving range, and this resulted in significant tendon damage on my elbow over a period of time, eventually leading to elbow surgery.

An RSI can seriously affect performance and, if not treated, could become a far more long-term injury. The common symptoms of this sort of injury are pain, weakness and fatigue that can become chronic, as well as numbness or swelling and restricted movement or altered mechanics.

Repeated movements might happen during training or even during daily activities. If you are a programmer, you type on your keyboard all day. If you are a long-distance runner, you keep landing on the same foot again and again, often for many miles and hours without a break. These movements lead to wear and tear that accumulates and often ends in an RSI. RSIs can also be the result of an imbalance caused by activities that only involve one side of the body—a tennis swing, writing, always lifting with one hand or even always letting your bag hang from the same shoulder. To the extent possible, loading both sides of the body equally reduces the chance of injury in the long run.

Treatment for RSIs begins with taking a break from the activity that caused the injury and resting the affected muscle, tendon or ligament. Application of ice and heat, as well as anti-inflammatory medication, might be used for milder RSIs, while physiotherapy and even surgery might be recommended for more severe cases. Ensuring that you warm up and cool down before and after exercise, and that you schedule adequate recovery in between training, can help reduce the likelihood of getting a repetitive stress injury.

In Summary

Keep in Mind

1. Despite being told that sitting is killing us, we did evolve to sit and save energy, when possible, evidenced in how hunter–gatherer communities still spend their days.
2. Exercise takes up the heart rate, strengthening the cardiac muscles and clearing the debris in the arteries; also increasing bone density and improving quality of sleep.
3. From the time we're children, we intuitively know how to run and instinctively enjoy it.
4. Exercise boosts levels of neurotransmitters and chemicals that, in turn, boost mood and brain development, while reducing stress. Working out can help improve mental health.
5. Regular cardio exercise lowers the resting heart rate, which is correlated with better health.
6. The repair of micro-tears in muscles caused by training leads to muscle strengthening, allowing them to adapt to further strain.
7. Mammals learn essential life skills while playing as infants, and there are many health benefits to be gained by playing a sport.
8. Sufficient recovery post-workouts can help maintain mobility and range of motion.
9. From swimming and running to HIIT, yoga and combat training, there are a variety of formats to choose from, based on your goals and preferences.
10. Periodization for high performance entails periods of high and low volume training, as well as phases for recovery and generalized training.

11. The perfectly chiselled six-pack abs or beach body might be less healthy than it looks, requiring less than 10 per cent body fat, which is particularly unhealthy for women.

12. The human body is capable of almost unimaginable feats of endurance and performance, that require mental and physical stamina and determination.

13. High physical performance comes with risks of overtraining and requires training under an experienced coach with sufficient recovery.

14. Recovery is crucial to maintain the body's internal balance or homeostasis. While there are several devices to track recovery, the best indicator is your own mood and body.

15. From foam rollers and saunas to ice baths and massages, we have a whole list of recovery options available.

16. Using the right form during workouts is essential to reap the benefits of exercise without injury.

17. Repetitive stress injuries occur when your workout or activity involves repeated movements and can become more serious if not treated immediately.

Take Action

1. If you sit for a large part of your day, try using a chair without a backrest or sitting cross-legged on the floor, and don't forget to take many breaks for small walks.

2. Don't be an 'active couch potato'. Incorporate as much movement in your life through daily activities as possible, such as by walking (instead of driving), gardening, carrying groceries.

3. Thinking about exercise as a fun or enjoyable activity, rather than a chore, can actually make you feel more motivated and your workout habit more sustainable.

4. If you're feeling a little stressed or anxious, try going for a brisk walk or run outdoors.

5. Before starting an exercise regime, make sure to consult a doctor and then work with a trainer who will first test your cardiovascular health before designing your workouts.

6. If your aim is to gain muscle while also losing fat, work with your trainer to create a regime that includes both resistance and aerobic training.

7. While strength training, if your workout is too light, the muscles don't adapt; while if it's too heavy, the body cannot fully repair muscles before the next session. The optimum adaptation occurs in sets of 4–6 reps using heavy weights.

8. If you used to play a sport as a child, get back on the field or the court—it's easy to use an app to find the nearest football field or badminton, tennis or table tennis court.

9. Work with a coach or trainer on improving your mobility and range of motion to ensure correct form and better recovery.

10. Use your devices and trackers to check in with your stats and recovery status, but don't forget to also check in with yourself—how you feel and what your mood is like.

11. Use the 'grip strength' test and the CO_2 tolerance test to see how well you've recovered from your last workout and whether you're ready for your next one.

12. If you don't have an ice bath machine or access to cryotherapy, try taking a really cold shower after a workout to gain some of the benefits of cold exposure.

13. Stretching and foam rolling after an intense workout can help prevent stiffness and stimulate quicker recovery.

5

SLEEP

Sleep is the best meditation. —Dalai Lama

As much as I'd hoped that my first visit to the ER would be my last, it was not meant to be. Perhaps, some health lessons must be learnt the hard way. In 2011, I was as busy as the next entrepreneur, working long hours, travelling, and putting all my energy into my start-up, Myntra. At the time, I had to travel to the US once every few months for very short trips of four or five days each. Travelling the twelve or thirteen-hour time zones twice in the span of five days was no joke, and I would struggle to fall asleep for the few days after landing in the US, as well as on my return to India. Assuming that this was a necessary side effect of work travel, I didn't think too much about it.

But after one of these trips, I just couldn't sleep. I went a whole day and a night without getting even a wink of sleep, and before I knew it, forty-eight hours had passed. By this time, I was exhausted and frustrated, and my brain felt foggy. I couldn't even think straight, and it soon reached a point where I could barely walk. Desperate to sleep, I decided to go to the ER again. I was given an injection and passed out right there on the ER bed for seven hours straight. I woke up feeling better and was referred to a psychiatrist, who gave me a prescription for sleeping pills, as well as detailed instructions on finding better ways to manage my sleep when I travelled abroad.

This experience terrified me but it made me take my sleep seriously for the first time in my life. I began to read everything I could about sleep and time zones, and my research, combined with some experiments on myself, helped me gain a much deeper understanding of how sleep forms the bedrock of any pursuit of good health. I now make sure to sleep as much as I can on a flight. As soon as I reach my destination, I try to spend one or two hours outdoors, getting some sunlight, which helps the body clock reset faster. If I need to, I take some sleep medication on the first or second day, as well as on my return, to help me adjust to the time zone. I avoid alcohol while travelling, and I make sure that I don't work out until I feel well rested.

Sleep is so integral to the human experience, that we spend a full third of our lives asleep. But sometimes, we forget about the sheer joy of sleep—letting go of the worries of the day, curling up in a calm and sheltered space, and waking up refreshed and ready to take on the day. I've come to realize that sleep is really one of the luxuries of life, an essential part of our health and wellbeing. Sleep is also one of those keystone habits that has a massive ripple effect on many other health habits. These days, the first thing I do when I wake up is check my Oura and Whoop device scores that give me detailed analyses of the previous night's sleep, and I am able to calibrate my plan for the day accordingly. Sleep is one of those investments that gives back in a major way—with increased vitality, vigour and high productivity throughout the day.

* * *

A quote often attributed to Benjamin Franklin, 'There will be sleeping enough in the grave', might have been misinterpreted by all those who use it as a grandiose statement against sleep. What was meant to be a warning against the dangers of being lazy, has instead become the slogan of those who brag about being able to survive on barely any sleep, as if this were a heroic feat. Luckily for us, this idea and the approach to sleep are changing, with several real life heroes of our time, including Federer and Tom Brady, emphasizing the importance of sleep for health.

For a long time, even after science began to unravel the mysteries of the human body and mind, sleep remained an enigma. It was believed that sleep was a period of inactivity, during which the body and the brain remained dormant, due to the lack of stimulation in the darkness of night. It wasn't considered a very interesting research topic, beyond the role of dreams and dream interpretation that grew popular in some circles. It was only in the 1950s that research into the field really picked up, with the discovery of REM, or rapid eye movements, during sleep. The first study, that recorded brain activity and eye movement patterns through the night, was conducted by Dr Nathaniel Kleitman, called the father of modern sleep research, at the University of Chicago. This led to studies of sleep disorders, eventually revealing deep connections between the quality and quantity of sleep and good health.

SLEEP: A NO-BRAINER

While sleep research has always focused on its neurological basis and effects, recent studies find that sleep might have evolved even before the brain did. In 2020, a team of scientists in Japan and Korea published a paper on their discovery that the simple hydra, a tiny organism that does not have a brain, sleeps. This was the culmination of several years of research that had not made it into the mainstream— whether simple organisms, such as invertebrates, sleep or not. Starting with cockroaches, studies had moved on to scorpions, fruit flies, and even the Cassiopeia jellyfish, which doesn't have much of a nervous system, discovering a behavioural basis for sleep. It seems all these creatures underwent periods of dormancy that were different from rest, and theories now suggest that sleep might play an important metabolic role. All of this points to the fact that sleep didn't evolve with the brain, and that it might date back to over a billion years ago. It also turns out that even hydra, like humans, suffer the ill effects of sleep deprivation on health!

Sleep has a profound impact on the body and mind—affecting everything, from appetite and heart health to productivity and focus. Just like eating and breathing, sleep is something our ancestors probably did without much fuss, and quite intuitively. However, our waking hours are so different from those of humans even a few thousand years ago, that our sleep has been affected, and not in a good way. We struggle to get to sleep, we struggle to wake up. We wonder how many hours of sleep we can get by on and contemplate the effectiveness of naps. And, of course, we turn to technology and supplements to track our sleep and to improve it. And, when all else fails, we try to sleep on it! In this section we'll try and gain some perspective on sleep—why it's important, how it works and how to get better at it.

THE ULTIMATE RECOVERY TOOL

When it comes to recovery, sleep might be the single most powerful tool we have. And guess what? It's free! If you train hard and don't sleep enough, it's unlikely that you will find any other method to make up for the recovery you're losing out on at night. Getting a good night's rest can be the ultimate game-changer when it comes to your recovery, unlocking potential you might not even have known existed within you.

What exactly happens while we sleep is still being investigated, but we now know that the brain is very active during this period of apparent inactivity. The brain at night is busy with housekeeping—cleaning up and repairing itself to prepare for further stimulation and engagement.

We sleep in roughly ninety-minute cycles, during which our brain waves go through four distinct phases. Most modern sleep tracking devices record these cycles by the minute and present a nifty chart in the morning for you to marvel at your performance or rue the missed chance of rejuvenating your mind and body.

One of the most important roles that sleep plays is in the synthesis and consolidation of memories. We spend the day processing numerous inputs from our environments, practicing new skills or absorbing new information. But we are also inundated with a huge amount of extra information that may never be relevant again. Based on our emotional reaction to various stimuli, the brain filters out unwanted information, while organizing long term memory which is critical for learning.

Another important function that the brain undertakes at night is the repair of wear and tear and the clearing of toxins from the body and brain, that accumulate as by-products of biological processes. Studies show that people who are chronically sleep deprived have higher levels of toxins in the body and take much longer to recover from injuries and infections. Compromising on the quantity and quality of the sleep we get prevents us from tapping into the deep healing powers of the brain, the legacy of millions of years of evolution.

One of the ways in which sleep plays a role in recovery is through the release of hormones in certain stages of sleep, specifically the human growth hormone (HGH) and testosterone, which play an important role in the repair of tissues, as well as in muscle and bone growth. Given that intense exercise, as we know, causes micro-tears in the muscle, it's clear that this repair mechanism is absolutely crucial for recovery. One study found that when sleep was restricted to only five hours a night in healthy young male subjects, their levels of testosterone dropped by 10 to 15 per cent in just one week. The increase in hormones happens during stage 3 or N3 of non-REM (NREM) sleep, when blood flow to the muscle tissues increases due to very low levels of brain activity. This stage of restorative sleep is also associated with a deep relaxation of the muscles, which could, in turn, relieve tension and symptoms of chronic pain.

In addition to slowing down the body's self-repairing process, sleep deprivation is also found to adversely affect immunity, while making the body more susceptible to injury. For example, one study hypothesized that athletes who are sleep deprived are at risk for musculoskeletal injury, as a result of lowered levels of growth hormones and increased cortisol that all affect protein pathways important for muscle health. Sleeping for recovery, therefore, doesn't just help fix some of the damage that training might have wrought, but also makes you more resilient for your next training session.

Sleep is also very closely related to the hormones that control our appetite. Studies have found lower levels of leptin (the hunger suppressing hormone) and higher levels of ghrelin (the hormone that stimulates appetite) in subjects who were sleep deprived[1]. Those who consistently sleep less than the recommended hours per night are also found to be more prone to obesity with higher BMI (body mass index). Not only does a lack of sleep increase appetite, it also seems to give us very specific cravings for high calorie foods[2].

So, if you've ever been the kind of person who thinks of sleep as wasted, unproductive time that you could have used to train or get fitter instead, it's time to think again. Sleep, in fact, can fill in all the gaps to help you achieve your health goals.

HEALTH HACK #13: Take the Perfect Nap

The ideal time for a nap is between ten and twenty minutes—five is too short to get its benefits, while longer than thirty minutes will leave you feeling groggy. Try and schedule a nap in the first half of the day, or post-lunch to coincide with the natural dip in energy. And remember, if you nap too late, you might find it harder to sleep at night.

THE SCIENCE OF SLEEP

Circadian Rhythms

Despite all the advances in technology and the number of apps and devices we have at our fingertips, the most sophisticated mechanisms sometimes exist in nature. One such is the circadian rhythm, often referred to as the body's internal clock. The word is derived from the Latin *circa*, meaning 'about' or around' and *dies* meaning 'day'. In humans, and in most animals and plants, the circadian rhythms of the body cycle approximately every twenty-four hours, and this relates directly to the rotation of the earth on its axis, leading to day and night. This biological clock helps determine our wakefulness and sleepiness, but also affects appetite, mood, body temperature, the release of hormones and metabolism.

While our internal circadian rhythms seem to stay fairly constant, they are helped along by external cues and stimuli, from sunlight to mealtimes, temperature to sleep patterns, and even regularly timed social interactions (a 4 p.m. coffee break with colleagues, or an evening walk with neighbours). These clues are known as 'zeitgebers', and the more we have, the more synchronized our circadian rhythms can be.

Biologically speaking, the circadian rhythm is governed by the suprachiasmatic nucleus, located in the middle of the brain, just above where the optic nerves intersect—the perfect spot to use information coming from the eyes. One of the many processes that this little bundle of neurons controls is core body temperature, that rises in the morning, peaks in the afternoon, drops around bedtime and reaches its lowest point about two hours after going to sleep.

Everyone's sleeping and waking cycles are slightly different, and this is because we experience peaks and troughs at different times. For example, about 40 per cent of the population are larks, meaning that they hit their peak early in the day, while 30 per cent, known as owls, experience their highs later in the day, and therefore might sleep and wake later than larks. The remaining 30 per cent are sort of in between morning and evening people. This tendency to be a morning person or an evening person is called your chronotype and is influenced by genetics.

Besides the suprachiasmatic nucleus, there is one other element that exerts influence over our circadian rhythm, and that is melatonin, also known as 'the hormone of darkness' and even 'the vampire hormone'. It is released by the pineal gland into the bloodstream soon after dusk, acting as a messenger, informing the brain and body that night is falling. Levels of melatonin start reducing during sleep, and at dawn, the pineal gland 'shuts off', and the absence of melatonin indicates that it is morning.

Unfortunately, there are some things that interfere with our natural circadian rhythms, most notably jetlag. When you travel to a different time zone, your suprachiasmatic nucleus could take up to one day for every hour of time difference, to adapt to the new zone. Fortunately, melatonin supplement pills are available, that could help you adjust more quickly to the change. Apart from travel and jet lag, shift work and sleep disorders can also affect the functioning of circadian rhythms. When the body's biological clock is interrupted in any way, it can have adverse effects on everything from mood to immunity to metabolism. In addition, the chronic use of artificial lighting and the light from screens can also play havoc with our sleeping cycles, which is why many of the tips we will look at later in this chapter will address these elements.

In 2018, researchers found that even our mitochondria function in response to this internal biological clock. Interruptions in the functioning of the circadian rhythm could negatively affect the levels of energy produced by the cells of the body.

Sleep Cycles

We all follow a pattern of sleep when we rest at night, shifting through stages that are associated with varying brain waves, eye movement activity and muscle activity. Sleep is broadly divided into NREM and REM sleep. Brain activity during REM sleep is very similar to that of wakefulness, and it is a time of vivid dreaming. REM sleep is also characterized by low muscle tone. NREM sleep has been further divided into three stages, known as N1, N2 and N3. Stages 1 and 2 are classified as light sleep, while 3 is the deepest sleep of the night; a period during which it is extremely difficult to wake someone up.

The length of a human sleep cycle is approximately ninety minutes, and on a typical night we go through about five cycles. The nature of the cycles changes through the night, however, as we spend most of the ninety minutes in the first half of the night in deep NREM sleep, and, later in the night, we shift to spending most of the cycle in REM sleep. This might be why you often wake up clutching onto the fragments of a dream that you were immersed in during the wee hours of the morning. This is also why cutting short your seven to nine hour rest by waking up several hours early means that you lose about a quarter of your sleep, but almost all of your REM sleep. If you're using a sleep tracker, you should ideally be spending 20–25 per cent of the night in REM sleep.

SLEEP STAGE	CHARACTERISTICS	MUSCLE TONE	BRAIN WAVES
Stage 1 NREM or N1	Lightest stage between wakefulness and sleep	Muscles active, leading to twitching	Shift from beta & gamma to alpha & theta waves
Stage 2 NREM or N2	Awareness decreases, we spend most of the night here	Muscle activity gradually decreases	Theta, with bursts of sigma waves known as sleep spindles
Stage 3 NREM or N3	Deep sleep, when breathing, heart rate, blood pressure and brain activity drop	Muscle atonia or paralysis	Delta waves or slow waves
REM or Stage 4	Movement of the eyes behind closed lids and lucid dreams	Very low muscle tone	Brain waves resemble waking state

Each stage of sleep is associated with certain benefits.

Light sleep in stage 2 of NREM is associated with improving the brain's capacity to learn or remember facts. The more sleep spindles, or bursts of electrical activity, there are in this stage, the better the learning ability. This happens through the transfer of memories from short-term to long-term storage, supposedly 'emptying' the short-term holding space for more learning. Deeper stages of NREM correspond with better memory retention. In one study, researchers first got subjects to learn a list of facts, and then allowed them to sleep only for the first half of the night (which we know is rich in NREM sleep) or only for the second half of the night (which is spent mostly in REM sleep). Those who spent the most time in deep NREM sleep, by sleeping in the first half of the night, were better able to remember the facts they'd learnt. NREM sleep has also been found to be absolutely crucial in the learning and perfecting of motor skills, whether playing the piano or a sport.

During REM sleep, our brains make unique connections, synthesizing varied sources and types of information, thus boosting our creativity. The REM sleep stage also plays a role in learning, memory and mood. Most significantly, babies and infants spend a great deal of their sleep in REM, from which it has been inferred that this stage plays an important role in brain development. During REM sleep, there is heightened activity in the visual, motor, emotional and autobiographical regions of the brain, and lower levels of activity in areas associated with rational thought. One study has found that good quality REM sleep lowers the levels of fear-related brain activity, particularly in the amygdala and hippocampus.

HEALTH HACK #14: Chamomile

Chamomile is one of the oldest herbs known for its medical properties, and was used in ancient Egypt, Rome and Greece, among other parts of Europe. Containing terpenoids and flavonoids, chamomile is thought to have anti-inflammatory, anti-cancer and several other health promoting properties, including calming the mind and body before sleep. Chamomile is best consumed as a freshly brewed tea.

What's Your Chronotype?

Our society has been designed as if we are a population of morning people. But if you look around at bleary-eyed teenagers trying to stay awake at the breakfast table before heading to school, or crowds of people downing coffees on their way to work, you'll realize this is simply not true. In fact, while the world seems to celebrate larks—those cheery morning types—the fact is that not being a morning person doesn't make you lazy. Each of us has a chronotype, a genetically programmed inclination to sleep and wake at certain times of the day, which, in turn, determines when we are at our most productive or energetic. While most of us can change the time at which we go to bed or wake up to suit the schedules enforced by our places of study or work, the fact is that we might not be at our best when we're not working in sync with our natural tendencies.

Dr Michael Breus, a clinical psychologist and a sleep expert, has classified four sleep chronotypes. A majority of people are Bears—they sleep and wake with the sun, are most productive mid-morning and face a slump in the mid-afternoon. Bears tend to be social and efficient creatures. Lions—most often type-A personalities—wake up early and might have several productive hours before lunch, but their energy wanes by the evening. On the other end of the spectrum is the Wolf chronotype, who struggle to wake early, and are most productive in the afternoon and again late in the evening. Creative people who are slightly introverted tend to be Wolves. The last chronotype is the Dolphin, who don't necessarily have a fixed sleep routine, but are light sleepers and struggle to fall asleep. Dolphins tend to be productive between mid-morning and early afternoon, but are often running on too little sleep.

Knowing that there exist among us such a variety of chronotypes is a good starting point to question the early mornings that most people are subjected to, from a very young age. By forcing people out of bed earlier, we aren't improving productivity, but adversely impacting health. We will look at the effects of sleep deprivation in detail shortly, but they range from depression, obesity and PCOD to the increased use of alcohol and tobacco. Teenagers—who experience a shift in their chronotypes as they mature and tend to sleep later—might be among the worst affected by routines skewed in favour of morning people. Some schools in the US have experimented with slightly later start times and have seen dramatic results. School districts in Minnesota, that changed the first bell from 7.25 a.m. to 8.30 a.m., reported improvements in attendance, test scores, mental health and overall behaviour. Some of the schools even reported fewer car crashes, one of the leading causes of death in older teens. All it took was an extra hour of sleep.

Another group of people who struggle with discrepancies between their chronotypes and their schedules are shift workers. In fact, the WHO recently classified shift work as a carcinogen. Often, factories and plants require staff on site 24X7 and, in order to be 'fair' to everyone, rotate employees on different shifts, sometimes within the same week. One of the most important aspects of better sleep health, however, is maintaining a regular routine. By eating, sleeping and waking at the same time every day—or at least five to six times a week—we can be in better control of our biological clocks. A study was conducted at a steel plant in Germany, where workers rotated between morning, evening and night shifts every two days. The researchers identified three broad chronotypes— early chronotypes, late chronotypes and intermediate chronotypes, and abolished the night shift for early chronotypes and the early morning shift for late chronotypes. Synchronizing workers' shifts with their chronotype led to employees reporting better sleep quantity and quality, and better wellbeing at work.

Changes to school schedules and increased flexibility in work timings are simple ways of helping people live in sync with their internal clocks. You can make changes in your own routine to make sure you're performing at your best, whether at work or workouts. Try and identify your chronotype and see if you can slightly tweak your schedule to get even a couple of extra hours of sleep—and discover the benefits to your health and productivity.

Setting Up the Sleep Environment

When it comes to sleep, there are many small changes you can make to have a big impact on the quality of your night-time rest. Among those changes is creating an environment that is conducive to a good night's sleep. Matthew Walker, a professor of neuroscience, whose research has focused on the science of sleep, suggests sleeping in a dark, cool, gadget-free bedroom for the best sleep. Removing every element that could be a distraction, from noisy clocks and bright lights to uncomfortable pillows and warm temperatures could help unlock the best sleep of your life.

Our sleep behaviour also changed thanks to the COVID-19 pandemic, especially in the early days of the lockdown. Interestingly, some people actually reported getting better sleep and sleeping longer, especially college students and night owls, who no longer had to wake up at the crack of dawn for classes and commutes. This group was probably in better sync with their circadian rhythms for the first time in their lives, thanks to no early alarms dragging them out of bed. For others, a lack of routine and exercise coupled with the stress and anxiety brought on by the virus robbed them of sleep, turning many into insomniacs and others into vivid dreamers.[3]

My own relationship with sleep these days has its ups and downs. On good days, I read before bed. Reading really calms my mind, which means I sleep at my scheduled time and manage to get a good night's rest so I can wake up ready for my workout. There are days, however, when I start watching something on Netflix, and before I even realize it, I've spent two or three hours binge-watching something so addictive that I can't stop. As a result, I don't sleep well or enough, miss my morning workout and fall into a vicious cycle. It's normal to have good days and bad days, but I find that having a routine and knowing what helps improve your sleep can help you get back on track.

Start by keeping your room free of gadgets that beep or blink, disturbing your rest. Thick curtains or blinds can help keep any artificial streetlight out of your room, while a dimmer mechanism for your ceiling lights, or lamps can keep the lighting soft at bedtime. At the same time, it's great if you're able to allow some natural morning light in to help wake you up, regulating your circadian rhythm. A 2014 study found that people who use e-readers with an artificial light before bedtime took an average of ten minutes longer to fall asleep and spent less time in REM than those who read a print book.

A room that's either too warm or too cold can also interrupt your sleep, so maintaining a constant temperature, that's on the cooler side, is ideal. While most recommendations for ideal sleep temperature vary from 18 to 20 degrees Celsius, in the Indian context that optimal number might be more like 21 to 23 degrees.

A comfortable mattress and pillow can make a big difference, as can the comfort and quality of your sheets and bedding. It might be worth investing in the best you can find if you want to transform your sleep and derive the many health benefits it offers. When it comes to sleep, even the littlest things matter. For example, having loud and bright colours or a cluttered room can interfere with the soft, calming environment you want to create. Choose delicate pastels for your bedroom and try to keep it neat to help you really get into the mood for a solid night's rest.

And finally, pay attention to the ambient sounds and smells in your room. Loud honking and traffic aren't exactly the lulling kinds of sounds you want to hear as you drift off. Soundproof windows, if that's an option for you, are worth the investment. Some people like to listen to calming sounds of nature before they sleep, while others like to have small water fountains that mimic the sounds of a babbling brook. Burning essential oils, like lavender, can also create a truly peaceful atmosphere that makes you sink gently and quickly into a good night's sleep.

Ancient Sleep

Not too long ago, productivity hackers—particular those in the Silicon Valley—were experimenting with polyphasic sleep, sleeping in very short bursts through the day. Some would only get one and a half or a few hours of 'core' sleep in a day, and make up for the rest in twenty-minute naps interspersed through the day. While there is little science behind this sleeping pattern and doctors warn of its health consequences, it turns out that historically, humans might not have been monophasic sleepers, and had a period of wakefulness in the middle of their night's sleep. There is evidence that right up to the sixteenth century, people had a 'first sleep' and a 'second sleep' interspersed by an hour of quiet activity at around midnight, during which they would read, pray with their family, do their chores or even sit around discussing their dreams. In hunter–gatherer societies, people took turns staying awake to keep an eye out for predators, and some tribal communities report two phases of sleep in the night even today.

FALLING ASLEEP

If only going to sleep were as easy as falling into bed and passing right out, instead of the uphill struggle it is for many of us. One of the most common sleep issues people encounter is the inability to fall asleep. Inevitably, when sleep fails to arrive after hours of trying, they reach for their phones and end up immersing themselves in a stimulating activity that only exacerbates the process. For some, the struggle to fall asleep can be a vicious cycle; a nightmare, if you will. Fortunately, it doesn't have to be this way. Simple bedtime routines and rituals can help you develop better sleep hygiene or habits. Start with shutting down all devices and avoiding electrical stimulation an hour before bed and eating your last meal at least two or three hours before, so digestion doesn't interfere with sleep onset. White light resembles morning light and signals the brain to wake, so it's a good idea to use yellow light in your bedroom and at night. Make sure you go to sleep at the same time every day. so that your circadian rhythm can settle into a predictable pattern. After switching off for the day, you could have a warm bath, listen to some soothing music, read a book, meditate or drink some herbal tea. Any activity you find relaxing, which doesn't stimulate your mind too much, is helpful—and when you develop these habits, your bedtime rituals will start signalling your brain to ready itself for restful sleep.

Given that we all have packed calendars, with barely any room to shift things around, it's important to ensure you keep aside a minimum of seven to eight hours for sleep, even if that means setting an alarm and excusing yourself from social gatherings. The idea that one can make up for lost sleep by sleeping in on Sundays or taking naps is a myth. Unfortunately, lost sleep is lost forever.

You might think of sleep as the opposite of exercise, and yet, the two are closely interrelated. This might sound familiar to you—the more often you work out, the more tired you feel, which makes it easier to go to sleep and easier to wake up and hit the gym in the morning. The converse is true too, of course: if you miss a workout, you might struggle to sleep until it's so late that there's no way you'll be able to wake up to exercise. A 2014 study[4] from the University of Georgia discovered that sleep problems were closely related to cardiorespiratory fitness. In another study[5], researchers from Northwestern University found that working out added an extra forty-five minutes of sleep for the participants who suffered from insomnia. They also found that delays in going to sleep resulted in shorter workouts the next day.

Many people boast about being resistant to the effects of coffee, but stimulants like caffeine and nicotine are notorious for their ability to interfere with your sleeping cycle. In fact, one study found that even a moderate dose of caffeine disrupted sleep, whether taken zero, three or six hours before sleep onset, compared to a placebo in the control. Perhaps as bad or even worse than caffeine is alcohol. Alcohol might have sedative effects initially, causing you to fall asleep quickly; however, it keeps you in light sleep and robs you of precious REM sleep. One 2013 study[6] found that alcohol at any dosage disrupts sleep in the second half of the night. Instead of caffeine or alcohol, a beverage that might help you fall asleep faster and lead you to a more restful night is hot chamomile tea, which is calming and relaxing. Warm milk is also part of many people's bedtime rituals.

To calm the overactive mind, Arianna Huffington recommends writing down every thought that might be worrying you or tasks that might need attention the next day, something she calls a mind-dump.[7] In addition, mindfulness or gratitude meditation can put you in a calmer and more relaxed frame of mind that makes it easier to fall asleep. A 2009 study[8] found that after a six-week mindfulness meditation course, participants fell asleep twice as quickly as they had before the training.

Hopefully, creating a ritual that works best for you will help to make bedtime something peaceful and calming that you look forward to, and less of a struggle that you dread each evening. Evolution has programmed us to spend nearly a third of our lives in the state of sleep, so we are all born champions of good sleep. As babies, we spend as many as eighteen hours every day sleeping, so we are clearly naturally very good at this until our lifestyle comes in the way. By adjusting your lifestyle, you can go back to being a naturally good sleeper and tap into one of the most nourishing biological faculties that we have at our disposal.

SLEEP DISORDERS

A ruffled mind makes a restless pillow. —Charlotte Brontë

Considering how important sleep is for the proper functioning of our minds and bodies, particularly for restoration, healing and health, it is unfortunate that many people suffer from a range of sleep disorders. In this section, we'll have a quick look at some of these—and review the key protocols and treatments to address these.

One of the most common sleep disorders is insomnia, in which you are unable to fall asleep, even when you give yourself the adequate time and the right environment in which to do so. Insomnia is categorized based on whether one has trouble falling asleep, known as onset insomnia, or staying asleep, which is maintenance insomnia. Chronic insomnia can lead to serious impairments in daytime attention and functioning and can also cause physical and mental health problems. The single biggest cause of insomnia is anxiety. This is related to an overactive sympathetic nervous system, keeping us in a chronic state of stress.

Narcolepsy is marked by excessive daytime sleepiness which can be extremely disruptive for health and productivity; sleep paralysis, which makes it impossible to move or talk when waking up; and cataplexy, which is a sudden loss of muscle control and could lead to a collapse. Most often, narcoleptic attacks are brought on by positive or negative emotions. Cataplexy resembles the muscle paralysis of REM sleep and is thought to be caused by an abnormality of the REM sleep circuitry in the brain. At the moment, there is no truly effective treatment for narcolepsy, and instead, its symptoms are managed with drugs like amphetamine and antidepressants.

It's likely that a third or half of the population over the age of thirty snores at night. If you've had a long, hard day, or a few drinks, it's likely you'll snore even more! The secret that most people are now privy to is that lying on your back increases the likelihood of snoring, and lying on your side reduces it—this is the case with positional snoring. Things get worrying, however, when it isn't just snoring that's a problem, but obstructive sleep apnoea, in which the airway actually closes off, affecting levels of oxygen. With sleep apnoea, the brain is deprived of oxygen for brief periods through the night and sleep itself is affected—you can barely reach the deeper stages of NREM sleep, as you keep waking up when you struggle to breathe, and it's unlikely you'll make it into REM. Sleep apnoea also affects blood pressure, weight, blood sugar and mood, increasing risk for heart attacks and strokes. The most common treatment for apnoea is continuous positive airway pressure (CPAP), a splint that props open the airway to prevent obstruction. Sometimes, losing weight and sleeping on your side can also address aponea, while, in some cases, oral devices or even surgery might be prescribed.

While sleep deprivation itself is not considered a disorder, it has been found to lead to profound disturbances in our health. In one study, controversial for the cruelty inflicted on the rodents, rats that were prevented from sleeping died within an average of fifteen days. In addition, if the rats were only prevented from getting into REM sleep, in a selective form of deprivation, they died almost as quickly as from total sleep deprivation. A deprivation of NREM sleep was also found to lead to death, although this took, on average, forty-five days. As a result of sleep deprivation, the rats lost body mass and they could not regulate their core body temperature, while their immune systems seemed to be failing. Postmortems showed that the rats suffered from fluid in the lungs, haemorrhaging, ulcers and physical shrinking of the organs, like the liver and kidneys. They had all died from septicaemia, a toxic bacterial infection tracing back to the rodents' own gut, that their immune system should have been able to fight off.

The conclusion that modern sleep medicine has come to is fairly straightforward—in the words of Matthew Walker, author of *Why We Sleep*, 'The shorter your sleep, the shorter your life.'[9] Poor quality of sleep and a lack of sleep have been associated with an increase in the risk for cardiac arrests. This happens due to increased heart rate and blood pressure as a result of sleep deprivation. Sleeping less than the adequate number of hours per night can lead to gaining weight and even obesity.

In a study mentioned by Matthew Walker in his book *Why We Sleep*, participants were put on two different sleep protocols—one of four nights of eight and a half hours of sleep, and another of four and a half hours of sleep. Each day, they were restricted to the same amount of physical activity and had access to food. It was found that the same participants ate 300 calories more each day when they were restricted to less than five hours of sleep a night![10] It's no wonder, then, that a lack of sleep is linked to weight gain. In fact, there is evidence that the obesity epidemic we face in our modern world is linked to the epidemic of sleep deprivation. In addition, studies have found that just one week of sleeping for less than four hours a night will result in a pre-diabetic state, wherein the body is 40 per cent less effective at absorbing glucose as it should be.

Sleep is absolutely essential for the smooth functioning of the immune system and for the body to heal itself. In one study conducted by Dr Aric Prather at the University of California[11], more than 150 healthy men and women were subjected to a sleep study for a week. After this, they were injected with a rhinovirus, the common cold virus. The team monitored the subjects the following week. The group was divided on the basis of how much sleep they'd had the previous week—less than five hours, five to six hours, six to seven hours and seven or more. The study found a clear linear relationship—the less sleep a participant had had, the more likely they were to catch a cold.

In the most sleep deprived group, the chances of catching the virus were 50 per cent, while in those who slept seven or more hours a night, the chances were just 18 per cent. As if all of this wasn't enough, sleep deprivation can increase your risk for

Alzheimer's, cancer, depression, hypertension and even erode your genetic make-up. A landmark study by Dr Derk-Jan Dijk[12] found that the activity of 711 genes was distorted after just one week of slightly reduced sleep. Genes linked to inflammation, stress and cardiovascular disease sped up their activity, while those related to stable metabolism and immunity, slowed down. Finally, a lack of sleep can also damage the telomeres of the chromosome, profoundly affecting our ageing process.

If you suspect that there might be something seriously wrong with your sleep and improving your habits by developing good routines doesn't help, sleep tests or studies offer a more detailed and accurate analysis.

SLEEP TRACKING

Tracking our sleep, something that was the domain of advanced medical practitioners in hospital settings not very long ago, is now easily done at home with the help of affordable devices. From using apps on your phone to the wearable Apple Watch and FitBit trackers, from devices to place under your mattress to more advanced wearable technologies, there are now many ways to gain insights into how well (or badly) we're sleeping. It's important to note, however, that not all of these are perfectly reliable because, unlike a sleep test in a hospital, they don't have a way of reading your brainwaves, and use other indicators to measure your sleep. The table below gives you a quick guide to various kinds of trackers and their advantages and disadvantages:

Level	How It Works	Pros	Cons
Basic— Smartphone Apps	Track movement & breathing while on the mattress at night; wake you up during light sleep	Easy to use & accessible—a great place to start	Not very accurate as results can be affected by sleeping partner, phones get overheated
Intermediate— Fitness Trackers	These devices use heart rate monitors to identify the sleep stage; Some have SPO2 sensors to gauge blood oxygen	Offer a great deal of data that can be compared against personal and average population statistics	The data, though detailed, is not completely accurate
Advanced— Wearables (Oura Ring)	The devices measure pulse, temperature & movement	Easy to wear, attractive to look at, highly advanced sensors with accurate data	

Almost all sleep trackers give you a sleep score, a metric that usually takes into account details like the number of hours of sleep logged, time taken to fall asleep, time spent in REM and NREM stages and time spent awake. This data is then measured against the averages of your gender and age, to give you a score between 0 and 100. In addition, many of the apps come with sleep coaches, personalized tips and ways of connecting your sleep with your overall health and fitness. Being able to analyse your sleep time in this much detail, seeing where you stand compared to the average and gaining insights into where you can do better, can all help you get your sleeping habits right back on track.

HEALTH HACK #15: Oura Ring

This tiny piece of technology worn on the finger tracks all kinds of body functions, giving you a whole bunch of statistics on your health. Its sensors track sleep in great detail, activity levels, calories, steps, heart rate, body temperature and even naps. All this with a tiny and beautiful ring! This truly feels like the future of health technology.

SLEEP SUPPLEMENTS & MEDICATION

Sometimes, even if we follow all the advice and tips for the perfect sleep environment, exercise regularly and eat right, we still might need a little extra help to improve our sleep quality. And that's where sleep supplements come in. Many of these are over-the-counter supplements, such as melatonin and magnesium, that help us get a better night's rest. In order to figure out the best supplement, when to take it and how much, it's a good idea to consult your doctor. In some cases, simple vitamin supplements might do the trick, while in others, a combination can help you get the perfect recipe for better sleep.

In extreme cases of insomnia and sleep disorders, where environmental and behavioural changes haven't worked, a doctor might prescribe sleeping pills. Most sleeping pills either help you fall asleep, help you stay asleep or both. Unfortunately, sleeping pills are not really the answer for getting a good night's rest (remember, there are no miracle cures!), and in fact, might end up doing more harm than good. The side effects of this medication vary from dizziness, headaches and gastrointestinal problems to prolonged drowsiness and impaired memory or performance during the day. When used for a short period of time to address a specific disorder, sleeping medication might work. However, in the long term it can lead to more serious issues of drug intolerance, drug dependence, withdrawal and rebound insomnia, in which the insomnia becomes even worse when you stop taking the pills.

A 2012 study published in the *British Medical Journal* found that the regular and long-term use of many types of sleeping medication were associated with a higher risk of death, as well as an increased risk for cancer. For these reasons, it's important to approach sleep medication with a healthy dose of wariness. If your doctor does prescribe them, first find out what your other options are and try making changes to your sleep hygiene before starting the pills.

POWER NAPS

A day without a nap is like a cupcake without frosting.—Terri Guillemets

Naps are no longer the domain of kindergarteners and babies. The term 'power nap' was coined by James B. Maas, to bring the supposedly 'childish' nap into a work setting. These days, napping is something even high performers recommend, while several companies have set up napping rooms at the office. While the question of whether naps can reverse the adverse effects of chronic sleep loss remains to be resolved, they have been found to be useful in addressing daytime sleepiness, which could be an outcome of sleep deprivation. The key is to plan and time your naps right to reap the benefits.

According to Chris Winter, author of *The Sleep Solution*, 'An early nap adds to the previous night of sleep but a late nap subtracts from the upcoming night of sleep[13].' Thus, in general, it's best to take a nap in the first half of the day, rather than the second half, which might make it harder for you to fall asleep that night. Most of us are familiar with the post-lunch drowsiness or slump. Many researchers believe this is the ideal time to schedule a nap, as it coincides with a natural feeling of daytime sleepiness. If you are an expert napper, you might also have noticed that the longer the nap is, the longer it takes you to snap out of the sleepy daze. And this is why the ideal length of a nap is twenty to thirty minutes. This ensures that you stay in stages 1 and 2 of light sleep, since waking up from deep sleep is much harder and leaves you feeling groggy (a state called sleep inertia). For best results, nap in a quiet, dark environment, and then expose yourself to sunlight straight after. If you can also get in a little movement, you will feel truly refreshed post-nap.

Napping has other benefits. A 2015 study by the Sorbonne University in Paris[14] found that brief naps of about thirty minutes could help release stress, while having a positive effect on the immune system. Other studies have corroborated the potential stress busting effects of catnaps. In addition, well-timed and executed naps have been found to have a positive impact on learning and creativity.

It seems that, with age, the benefits of napping only grow. Findings from the China Health and Retirement Longitudinal Study[15] found a positive correlation between post-lunch napping and improved cognition in older adults. Several other studies have found a similar effect on cognition, while also finding that napping improved the quality of sleep and reduced daytime sleepiness in older adults.

I hope this chapter has convinced you about the incredible benefits of a good night's sleep. If you want days filled with vitality, productivity at work and a life of learning and growing, without increasing health ailments, sleep has to be your foremost concern. Even if your modern life has eroded the quality of your sleep, the good news is that, with lifestyle changes and persistence, you can learn to be a good sleeper again. And once you get a taste of the immense rejuvenating and healing powers of great sleep, you will never look back!

IN SUMMARY

Keep in Mind

1. Sleep is crucial for memory processing, repair of wear and tear, hormone regulation and almost every other aspect of the body's function. Sleep deprivation negatively affects immunity and appetite, causing a host of chronic illnesses.

2. Our circadian rhythms remain fairly constant, helped along by external stimuli, but interrupted by jet lag and overexposure to artificial light.

3. We shift through four stages of sleep at night, each one associated with different effects on the body and the mind.

4. People have different chronotypes or times of the day at which they are more and less active and alert. Adjusting work shifts and school start times helps align this.

5. The COVID-19 pandemic changed the way we sleep in many ways—some of us slept better than ever, while anxiety and a lack of routine robbed others of a good night's rest.

6. Exercise in the day helps us sleep better at night, while a restful night of sleep makes us more likely to get to our workouts the next morning.

7. Sleep deprivation, though not a disorder like insomnia or narcolepsy, has negative consequences on health.

8. There are now many affordable devices to help track your sleep quantity and quality, helping you understand your sleep cycles and how you can get better rest at night.

9. Many over-the-counter supplements are excellent ways of supporting better sleep, and sleep medications, while effective, can be addictive and should be used with caution.

10. Naps might help relieve stress, while having a beneficial effect on the immune system.

Take Action

1. Change your relationship with sleep—it isn't time wasted, but time spent in the most important processes of recovery, memory formation and health preservation.

2. If you're flying internationally, try to take a daytime flight, avoid alcohol while travelling and try to get some morning sunlight at your destination.

3. Are you a bear, a wolf or a dolphin? Understand when you feel least and most energetic to figure out your chronotype and adjust your schedule accordingly.

4. For the best sleep, ensure your room is dark, cool and comfortable, free of disturbances from gadgets, blinking lights and noise.

5. Simple bedtime rituals, such as a cup of chamomile tea, a meditation session or listening to sleep stories on a podcast, can help you fall asleep better.

6. Avoid drinking caffeine after 4 p.m. so its stimulant effects don't interfere with sleep.

7. Struggling to sleep? Ask your nutritionist or doctor to prescribe over-the-counter supplements that could help you streamline your body clock and improve the quality of your sleep.

8. The best power naps are taken in the first half of the day and restricted to twenty to thirty minutes. These leave you feeling refreshed, without compromising on your night's rest.

6

BREATH & MEDITATION

Breath is the bridge which connects life to consciousness, which unites your body to your thoughts.—Thich Nhat Hanh

I have always been struck by how similar places of spiritual contemplation are to the natural surroundings we seek to find moments of calm. Temples, churches and mosques, for example, are usually vast spaces defined by a feeling of openness— beautifully lit with sunlight or a candle flame, with high ceilings and music in the form of ringing bells, chants or choral voices. The feeling evoked by these places isn't very different from what we experience when we are trekking in the mountains or walking in a forest or swimming in the open ocean. But instead of decorative ceilings, we have the open sky above us, and in place of music or candles, we have birdsong and the light of the sun and stars.

These sorts of multisensory experiences seem to inspire meditative states, inducing a deep sense of calm—allowing us to slow down, reflect, and observe ourselves. I recently visited Auroville, where I had the opportunity to meditate in the Matrimandir, and I experienced for myself, this state of quiet contemplation.

Auroville is a fascinating place—an experimental township set up in 1968 with the vision to establish a 'universal city', where people could live in peace and harmony as citizens of the world. Auroville does not subscribe to any political belief or creed, instead striving for true human unity. For many people in the 1960s and 1970s, this represented the radical freedom that the hippie culture aspired to—an escape from the confines of traditional society to pursue journeys of introspection for the greater good. The idea has drawn people from around the world and different walks of life—many who have given up lucrative careers to become part of the community—and the land occupied by Auroville, once dry and barren, is now a lush and serene forest.

At the heart of Auroville is a structure that defies description—some compare it to a lotus in bloom, others see a golden golf-ball-shaped object out of a sci-fi film. This is the Matrimandir, literally meaning 'temple of the Mother', built in accordance with the vision of the Mother, Auroville's founder and spiritual collaborator of Sri Aurobindo. The golden sphere rises from the ground, with an inner chamber crafted of pure white marble that is centred around a large crystal globe. The crystal captures a beam of sunlight that streams in from the top of the dome, illuminating the silent space that is dedicated to non-denominational meditation.

As I walked up to the Matrimandir, I was stuck by the serenity of the surroundings—the carefully designed gardens and the sprawling banyan tree casting its shade on one side. The first glimpse of the actual structure, which took almost four decades to build, is hard to describe—this glowing orbit emerging from the earth, with shimmering golden discs that are radiant as they reflect the sun.

Inside, the space is the very definition of silence. I had the opportunity to sit in the chamber for about an hour in quiet contemplation. There was a moment when I experienced a deep feeling of oneness—as if my sense of self merged with the space around me. As I sat there, I felt as if the little things in life—the stresses and worries of everyday living—melted away and seemed insignificant in comparison to what I was experiencing. This was a profound experience for me—one that has made me reflect upon the nature of meditation and its role in the health of both the mind and the body.

* * *

Breathing is truly the most constant thing in our lives—something we have all done every moment of every day for as long as we've been alive and will continue to do until we, literally, take our last breath. It is one of life's most essential processes and, arguably, the one that makes us living beings. We breathe approximately twenty-two thousand times every day and over 700 million times in our lifetime. It is something we do mostly unconsciously and wholly instinctively, right from the moment we take that first lungful of oxygen at birth. While we talk a lot about nutrition and fitness and, lately, even about meditation and sleep, when it comes to breathing, we seem to take for granted that we're doing it right.

Just as our eating, moving and sleeping habits have been affected by modern lifestyles, our breathing has been affected too. It isn't just the quality of the air we breathe, that has changed for the worse thanks to rising pollution in cities. It's also about how we breathe and how much we breathe. Everything, from stress and processed foods to sedentary jobs, constant stimulation and chronic lifestyle diseases, affects the way we breathe. These are things we likely give very little thought to and, perhaps, it's time we started taking our breath a little more seriously.

Breathing ensures that every cell of the body gets the oxygen it needs to function, while removing waste carbon dioxide created by metabolic processes. However, breath plays a much more important role than that. Think about the things we often say to people when they're stressed or upset: 'just breathe' or 'inhale, exhale'. This illustrates the incredibly powerful role that the breath plays to connect the mind and the body. Focusing on the breath is a key element of yoga, meditation and other ancient mind–body practices, and the way we breathe can alter our mental state, making our attention razor sharp or calming an anxious mind. Altering the rate and depth of your breathing can help you recover better during rest periods while you're working out and can boost your exercise performance.

It doesn't end there. Your breath influences not just your mental state, physical activity, focus and mood, but also your eating habits, sleep quality and overall wellbeing. Breathing right might just be one of the most simple and essential hacks to bring the rest of your health journey together. At the heart of almost every ancient health practice lies the breath, as evidenced by the feats of Indian yogis, Buddhist monks and Chinese martial artists. Our breath could hold the secret to healing, fighting ageing and achieving cutting-edge performance.

HEALTH HACK #16: Take a Breath

The way we breathe can either stress us out or help us feel relaxed and calm. Short, shallow breaths through the mouth can actually make us agitated, while slow, deep breaths through the nose can release tension. Try this: inhale for four counts, hold your breath for four counts, exhale for four counts and then hold your breath for another four counts. Do a few cycles of this for a sense of calm.

WHY BREATHING MATTERS

While the physiology of the breath was a mystery for a long time, varying theories existed—not scientifically accurate, but each recognizing the centrality of breathing to human existence. For the early Greeks, the breath was synonymous with ideas of the soul. Some believed that the soul was inhaled through the air and into the brain, while others pictured the soul residing as breath in the chest, as pneuma, the life essence.[1] Empedocles, a Greek philosopher and doctor in the fifth century B.C., explained breathing as an exchange of air through the pores of the skin. A theory that echoed this concept was put forward by Plato, who believed that an 'inner fire' forced air out through the nose, leaving a void that was filled by air absorbed into the body through the skin. In the second century A.D., Galen, a Greek doctor who was invited by Marcus Aurelius to be physician to the gladiators of Rome, was the first to identify the diaphragm and respiratory muscles in the anatomy of breathing. Even though his understanding of the process of breathing was far from accurate, his theory lasted until the seventeenth century, when oxygen was finally discovered and respiration, the way we now know it, was explained.

There is a Hindu belief that the length of one's life is determined at birth, defined by the number of breaths one has. The belief was that one's lifespan shortened with illness, stress or other conditions that quickened the breath. In this context, the idea of 'wasting your breath' takes on an entirely new meaning.

Ancient Indian and Chinese traditions have recognized breath as the vital life force, terming it 'prana' and 'qi' (pronounced 'chi') respectively. It is believed that this energy flows through all living beings, and a disruption in this flow causes illness. Modern science has validated this wisdom, though we may use different terms to describe it.

Each of our forty trillion cells requires oxygen to survive. The reaction between simple sugar and oxygen produces energy in the form of ATP, which powers all cellular processes. Carbon dioxide and water are the by-products of this chemical reaction, which are both also equally critical for survival.

The unique thing about the process of breathing is that it comes under both our conscious and unconscious control. If we pay attention to it, we can control the way we breathe, how deep or how long. But the moment we let go of that control, we still continue to breathe because the autonomic nervous system takes over. It is this unique nature of breathing that renders it so powerful. Because of its connection to our autonomic nervous system and because of our ability to control breathing, we can indirectly control our autonomic nervous system. It is no wonder that just by varying our breathing patterns, we can alter the state of our mind and body.

From ancient traditions to modern breathing protocols validated by science, we now have numerous breathing techniques that can have a powerful impact on health and performance. In this chapter we will gain a basic understanding of the science of breathing and various breathing protocols that you can consider incorporating in your health regimen. Almost all popular breathing practices include one or more combinations of three fundamental manipulations of the breath.

a. Fast: When we inhale and exhale faster than normal, we exercise our lung muscles. This is great for short bursts of energy, opening up the nasal passages and strengthening the lungs.

b. Slow: Slowing down our breathing to a rate of one breath per ten to fifteen seconds has a profound anchoring effect, requiring us to focus and calming us down. This also improves CO_2 metabolism in the body which is critical for many biological functions.

c. Hold: Periodically holding the breath for a few seconds up to a minute is a powerful way of improving the efficiency of breathing and improving stamina.

HEALTH HACK #17: *Pranayama*

The practice of breath control, Pranayama, is an integral part of the ancient practice of yoga. Early practitioners recognized the centring power of Pranayama and its effects, not only on calming the mind, but on the health of the body too.

The Science of Breathing

When we breathe, the first point of contact with the air we inhale is usually and preferably the nose. Tiny bones and hair-like cilia help trap particles, moisten and warm the breath, filtering it before it enters the windpipe that takes it to the lungs.

Breathing is the result of a beautiful coordination between a range of muscles, organs and molecules. Every time we inhale, the diaphragm, which is an umbrella-shaped muscle at the base of our lungs, contracts. This increases the volume of the thoracic cavity, and the negative pressure thus created draws air into the lungs. Each time we exhale, the diaphragm expands, decreasing the volume of the thoracic cavity and emptying the lungs of air. Unfortunately, most adults use only about 10 per cent of the diaphragm's range while breathing. You can test whether you are engaging the diaphragm by placing one palm on your chest and one on your abdomen, just below your rib cage. While breathing, the palm on your chest should barely move, while the one on your abdomen should rise and fall with inhalations and exhalations. Many breath techniques that teach breath holding and extended exhalations can improve diaphragmatic breathing—which is good practice when it comes to the breath.

An interesting thing about breathing is the involvement of the two branches of the autonomic nervous system. In case you need a quick refresher of high school biology, the autonomic nervous system consists of the nerves that control our body's unconscious processes. It is further divided into the sympathetic and parasympathetic nervous systems. When we inhale, the sympathetic branch, known to activate the fight-or-flight response, briefly speeds up our heart rate. When we exhale, we activate the parasympathetic nervous system which slows our heart rate and brings about a feeling of relaxation. When we breathe shallowly or hyperventilate, we activate the sympathetic nervous system and with it, the body's stress response. As you might know by now, a state of stress is not conducive to health or recovery. However, by focusing on deep diaphragmatic breathing, with longer exhalations, we trigger the parasympathetic nervous system and its relaxation response.

It is considered normal for a healthy person to breathe between twelve and twenty times a minute, drawing in about 500 ml of air with each inhalation. A higher breathing rate leads to a higher intake of air and, while you might think that more air can only be good for you, it can in fact lead to a host of problems. Many people who are exploring and pushing the boundaries of the science of breath claim that in fact one of the underlying causes of many chronic illnesses is this culture of 'over breathing'. Many of the ancient breathing practices from India, China and elsewhere focus not just on slowing down the breath, but also decreasing the amount of air inhaled.

Not only have we become chronic over breathers, we've also become chronic mouth breathers, and this could be among the main factors for many of the chronic illnesses and lifestyle diseases we now face.[2] The structures of the nasal cavity filter out pollutants, increase humidity of the air and convert its temperature to match that of the body. In addition, during nasal breathing, nitric oxide is formed in the sinuses and nasal passages, and being a vasodilator, this improves circulation and overall respiratory function, while also influencing immune and other essential functions. Oral breathing, on the other hand, tends to lead to chronic hyperventilation which can cause dizziness and the constriction of blood vessels, putting the body in a constant state of stress. Some dentists also believe that mouth breathing is the leading cause of dental cavities, having a stronger impact even compared to sugar consumption.

George Catlin was a portrait painter who spent much of his life documenting and studying the lives and cultures of over 150 Native American tribes between 1830 and 1860. In 1870, he published a book by a somewhat curious name: *Shut Your Mouth and Save Your Life*.[3] During his travels and interactions with these communities, he observed that every single one of them breathed through their nose, whether they were awake or asleep. He also noticed that they didn't suffer from many of the chronic ailments that plagued most people with a 'Western' lifestyle and had a markedly lower mortality rate in children under the age of ten. He believed that the way they breathed made all the difference. Catlin went on to talk about how mothers would press the lips of their babies closed after nursing them to make them breathe through their noses and, when babies were sleeping, would pinch their lips together if they were found breathing through their mouths.

Unfortunately, most of us now suffer from chronic nasal obstruction caused by stress, allergies, pollutants and other elements of modern life, making us mouth breathers by habit. James Nestor, the author of *Breath: The New Science of a Lost Art*, submitted himself to a study under Dr Jayakar Nayak[4] of the Rhinology department at Stanford, in which he spent ten days breathing only through his mouth as he went about his everyday life, and the next ten days breathing only through his nose.

During his week of mouth breathing, he struggled—his snoring increased by over 4,000 per cent, his sleep apnoea events became obstructive, his blood pressure spiked putting him into a hypertensive state, his heart rate variability dropped indicating a state of stress and his mental state was constantly fuzzy. When he began phase two of the study, in which he breathed exclusively through his nose, his blood pressure normalized almost immediately, his heart rate variability increased and the levels of carbon dioxide in his body went up. By the end of the experiment, he had no sleep apnoea events and his snoring came down drastically.

An understanding of the science of breathing can, if you choose, give you a superpower of sorts. Free diving is a sport involving diving into the depths of the ocean without any scuba gear or breathing apparatus. While most of us struggle to hold our breath longer than about thirty seconds, free divers can go several minutes without breathing. In fact, the last two world records for longest breath holds were held by free divers, although achieved in swimming pools rather than in the deep sea. The current record is held by Budimir Sobat, who, in 2021, held his breath for twenty-four minutes and thirty-seven seconds—a duration many journalists point out is longer than most sitcoms! What is interesting to note about freediving is that most people who have tried it will speak not about what their body went through, but how meditative or mind-expanding the experience was. In addition, while they learn techniques of holding the breath and how to calculate levels of oxygen and carbon dioxide in their bodies, the single most important skill is learning to control the mind. The physiological act of breathing tethers the body to the mind.

The other field in which control over the breath is a desirable skill is the world of magic and illusions. From Harry Houdini to David Blaine, the repertoire of famous illusionists has almost always included a breath holding trick, usually trapped into some sort of structure that is then placed underwater. While some say Houdini's famous underwater trick was a mere illusion, Blaine has talked about using free diving training techniques to prepare for his own.

FAINTING FOR BREATH

The image of the fainting woman in Victorian times is a familiar one, and it might actually be more than a sexist stereotype. Striving for hourglass figures with unnaturally tiny waists, women were often laced into corsets so tight that they could barely breathe. Thanks to this, it is believed they often fainted from a lack of oxygen, requiring smelling salts to revive them. It's a good thing that we eventually realized that breathing was more important than a woman's figure!

BREATHING & PERFORMANCE

Have you noticed your breathing when you do an intense workout or go for a long run? Are you a calm and collected nose breather, or do you find yourself quickly out of breath, opening your mouth and gasping for air like a fish out of water? When we exercise, there is an increased demand for oxygen in the body. In fact, you might sometimes find that your ability to exercise is limited not by muscle soreness or physical fatigue, but by an inability to continue breathing through a workout, which increases perceived exhaustion.

The body's ability to use oxygen depends on the levels of carbon dioxide, and this is why training the body to breathe less, slower and through the nose can actually improve aerobic endurance and stamina. This will increase levels of carbon dioxide, improve circulation and stimulate the absorption of oxygen by the muscles and tissues being used. Breathing less simulates the effects of high-altitude training—something many elite athletes do—as it boosts red blood cells and increases the oxygen being carried through the body.

In the 1990s, Dr John Douillard, who trained elite athletes including Billie Jean King, studied the effect of nasal breathing on performance on stationary bikes. He found that nasal breathing could reduce exertion by half, because the rate of breath came down drastically.[5] For example, while mouth breathing at high intensity, one athlete's breathing rate was forty-eight breaths per minute, which came down to just fourteen breaths per minute during nasal breathing. While breathing orally, athletes ended up panting through their mouth and struggling to catch their breath. Levels of perceived exertion were also significantly lower during nasal breathing exercise.

If you're a mouth breather during exercise, shifting to nasal breathing might at first feel uncomfortable and even difficult. Your first instinct will be that you feel like you're suffocating or not getting enough oxygen. But if you were to connect yourself to a pulse oximeter, you'd find that the oxygen levels actually remain steady. You'll also find that you can slowly push yourself to improve, running or cycling longer distances on fewer and slower breaths, with less air. Thus, you will be gaining in efficiency.

While exercising, a focus on the breath is important. If you've ever practiced yoga, you will know that the breath acts as a centring force, and every posture is tied to an inhalation or exhalation. Similarly, many runners practice a pattern of breathing to keep a rhythm with their pace. For example, the 2:2 pattern requires taking two steps while inhaling and two steps while exhaling. During strength and conditioning sessions, you might have heard your trainer telling you to exhale on the exertion and inhale in between reps.

In addition to finding a rhythm that will keep you focused on your performance, it's also important to breathe the right way. Unfortunately, a lot of us interpret a deep breath as a big gasp of air through the mouth that expands the chest. However, the most important element of breathing right is to engage the diaphragm, which activates the core and expands the abdomen. This form of deep breathing ensures that your blood is well oxygenated, so oxygen reaches all your muscles. The other thing to remember is to focus on the exhalation as much as on the inhalation, keeping it slow and long. In fact, instead of the 2:2 pattern, you might want to try something more like 2:4, with an exhalation that's twice as long as the inhalation. This too might feel slightly uncomfortable at first, but gradually, you will notice improvement reflected in your endurance or distance.

Knowing the pivotal role of the breath in performance, you can try some of the techniques that we cover later in the chapter or do your own research and experiments to find out what works best for you.

BREATHING BETTER

While the role of breath in health, performance and recovery might sound novel to us, the fact is that ancient cultures were practicing and perfecting the art of breath millennia ago. In fact, there are inscriptions dating back to the Indus Valley civilization 5,000 years ago that depict a person in a yoga pose, practicing a belly breathing technique. Drawing on these traditional formats as well as on cutting-edge science, there are various techniques and methods to practice better breathing for better health.

In India, many of us are familiar with Pranayama, the yogic practice of breath awareness. Some of the common Pranayama techniques are *nadi shodhana* (alternate nostril breathing), *sitali* (to cool the body and calm the mind), *ujjayi* or ocean breath (done while constricting the throat to make a sound like the waves) and *kapalabhati* or skull shining breath (forceful exhalations), among others. Pranayama is found to lower blood pressure in hypertensive patients, resulting in reduced stress, better mood and lower cortisol levels, leading to better cardiovascular health.[6]

The Wim Hof method of breathing involves lying down with the eyes closed and alternating between controlled hyperventilation or deep, quick and forceful inhalations in short and powerful bursts and holding the breath for as long as possible. This technique is best done after consulting with a doctor, and should not be practiced while driving, swimming, standing up or in the shower. This is a form of controlled hyperventilation that is used by Wim Hof to take control of his autonomic nervous system as well as immunity, which, he says, improves overall health.

One of the simplest yet most powerful techniques is known as box breathing. While lying down or sitting comfortably, you start by exhaling for four counts, then hold your breath with your lungs empty for four counts, inhale for four counts and hold the breath in your lungs for four counts. You can also visualize the four sides of a box, changing colour one by one in tandem with the four steps of the breath.

Strength and conditioning coach Brian Mackenzie recommends two tests to see where you stand when it comes to your breath. For the first, take a deep breath and exhale slowly. At the end of the exhalation, time yourself to see how long it takes until you need to breathe in again, without pushing yourself too hard. Ideally, you should be able to last thirty seconds. The second test requires you to take a deep breath and then exhale as slowly as you can to see how long you can spend exhaling. According to Mackenzie, you should be able to spend a full minute exhaling from one deep breath.

The great thing about breath exercise is that it is readily accessible anytime, anywhere and you can practice it for any duration you like. Even one deep exhalation or one slow, measured breath might help you get anchored and feel renewed as you continue to deal with the challenges of your day.

HEALTH HACK #18: Dhyana

In what might appear as the perfect union of the ancient and the modern, the Dhyana ring is a device that tracks your meditation sessions. Based on heart rate variability, Dhyana gives you feedback on how you did on three parameters— breathing, relaxation and focus—while measuring how many minutes of actual mindfulness you experienced. A sleek device that syncs to an app on your phone might be your answer to becoming a better meditator.

WHAT IS MEDITATION

For a long time, meditation was considered the domain of monks, ascetics, priests and yogis—something that involved sacrifice and renunciation, on the solitary path to nirvana. It was shrouded in mystery and spirituality. After it travelled to the West and came to be associated with celebrities like The Beatles, Mia Farrow and, more recently, with top athletes and Silicon Valley executives, meditation has grown increasingly popular. Over the last few decades, its practices have been validated by cutting-edge science and rigorous research, making it a tool for every performance and health seeker's arsenal.

The immense positive impact of meditation is incredible, given how little time is needed to practice it. Experienced monks may meditate for hours at a time, but for most of us, just a few minutes a day can do wonders. I strongly urge you to consider making meditation an integral part of how you live your life, and you will not regret it.

What exercise is to the body, meditation is to the mind, cultivating greater awareness, focus and relaxation. The goal of meditation is to develop a calm mind that is aware of the present moment and the self, without judgement or expectation. Meditation offers the opportunity to realize the value of the present and to learn how to wholly experience every moment.

Meditation is one of those things that can be incredibly simple and accessible, and yet, can also be one of the most challenging practices. All you really need is a quiet corner and as few as ten minutes of your time. There are a host of guided meditation apps, classes at local gyms and even online sessions. You can choose to begin with as few as two minutes of meditation a day or start with ten and gradually work your way up. Most beginners' meditation sessions involve a focus point—either the breath, a visualization, an object or a chant of some sort.

The essence of meditation is developing the self-awareness to notice when the mind shifts away from its focus or gets distracted and the habit of gently guiding the mind back to the present moment. This is, at once, an effortful and effortless practice, requiring close attention, while remaining in a state of relaxed awareness. It can be uncomfortable and frustrating, but the important thing is to be kind and patient with yourself and to be consistent. It's okay to have a mind that wanders, and it's only natural to be distracted. You might feel restless or sleepy or struggle to focus, and that's okay. What is important is to return to the practice, again and again. In a world where there is stimulation from every direction at every moment of the day, it's important to learn how to quiet the 'monkey mind' and to focus on the present, instead of worrying constantly about the past and the future. Meditation might just be the key to unlocking true health.

THE SCIENCE OF MEDITATION

Meditation might be based on some of the most ancient philosophies and traditions, and yet, it has become a favourite subject of modern science. One of the earliest studies was conducted by B.K. Anand, considered the founder of modern neurophysiology in India, in 1961. It was reported that he had 'found that yogis could meditate themselves into trances so deep, that they didn't react when hot test tubes were pressed against their arms'.[7] Since then, there have been numerous scientific investigations into how meditation affects the body and the brain, with some encouraging results.

One of the important ways in which meditation impacts our overall health is by changing the way we perceive or are affected by stress. Stress is closely linked to inflammation which is at the root of almost all modern chronic lifestyle diseases. Studies have shown that experienced meditators have lower levels of cortisol, lower perceived stress and a smaller inflammatory response to stress than non-meditators. Meditation has been found to lead to greater resilience to stress and improved feelings of wellbeing. This healthier response to stress by meditators has been linked to dampened reactivity in the amygdala, which also brings about a greater sense of emotional stability. This could mean that meditation might play a role in protecting us from or reversing illnesses related to chronic stress and inflammation.

In one of the few longitudinal studies of meditation, neuroscientist Clifford Saron conducted a battery of tests on participants who were doing a three-month long meditation retreat. The meditators spent six hours a day meditating, and the control group were those who had signed up for the course but were still on the waitlist. The participants, who were tested at the beginning, middle and end of the course, reported less anxiety, greater overall wellbeing, better resilience in the face of emotional upsets and a freedom from impulses—all results that persisted in a follow-up test, five months after the retreat.

In their book, *Altered Traits: Science Reveals How Meditation Changes Your Mind, Brain and Body,* authors Daniel Goleman and Richard Davidson put forward the idea that the profound changes brought about by a long-term meditation practice reflect actual alterations in brain function. Meditators seem to have trained certain parts of the brain to make them less reactive to stress, less anxious and more able to stay present and fully attentive in the moment. In his lab, Richard Davidson has measured hundreds of yogis with lifetime meditation hours ranging from 10,000 to over 60,000. One of the telltale signs of a lifelong meditator is the strong and permanent presence of gamma waves, that are associated with a feeling of connectedness and heightened awareness—much like those we experience when awed by a performance, nature's beauty or a moment of insight. This is the strongest scientific validation yet of the underlying neurobiological signature brought about by meditative practices.

The tendency of experienced meditators to react less negatively to negative or stressful situations has been linked to a stronger connectivity between the prefrontal cortex, that manages our reactivity, and the amygdala, which triggers the fight-or-flight response. Advanced and seasoned meditators don't just experience a dampened amygdala response to stressful situations but have stronger operative connectivity between these two regions of the brain. It appears that by meditating regularly, one learns to take active control of the prefrontal cortex, thus quieting the amygdala and its effects.

Increasingly, an integrated approach, which includes meditation practice, is being taken to address the symptoms of mental illness. While researchers are still cautious about overstating the relationship between meditation and improved mental health, studies have shown mindfulness-based meditation can help alleviate the symptoms of anxiety and depression to a moderate extent. In addition, research has also discovered that even in ageing populations, meditation can have a positive effect on cognition, particularly on memory and attention, which can help delay the onset of cognitive decline and age-related disorders.

Studies continue to explore the varied positive impacts that meditation could have on health through its holistic mind–body method. There is some evidence of its role in improved sleep, management of chronic pain and even in healthier relationships. While meditation might not be a replacement for conventional therapies, especially in the case of chronic and serious ailments, its use as a complementary form of treatment is definitely worth exploring.

If all this evidence of neural strengthening still hasn't convinced you, maybe these findings will—meditation might make the brain grow and it might also help you to live longer. A meta-analysis of brain imaging studies of meditators found that several parts of the brain might grow in response to meditation, among them the insula, responsible for emotional self-awareness; the somatic motor areas that sense touch and pain; and regions of the prefrontal cortex involved in attention and meta-awareness.[8]

In 2016, a UCLA study found that meditation might slow down the age-related shrinking of the brain. Among the participants, those fifty-year-olds who had been long-term practitioners had brains that appeared 7.5 years younger than those of non-practitioners of the same age.[9] All these studies, however, still don't quite distinguish between the different types of practice and the intensity at which they are practiced, so this evidence is still a work in progress. However, there's enough to show that there are immense benefits for our brain!

So, we not only have a whole variety of meditation practices to choose from, but we also have very strong scientific evidence validating the positive impact of the practice. If the pursuit of good health is important to you, you have no excuse at all but to incorporate a meditation practice in your life. It can be as simple as mindful breathing or focusing on something for a few minutes, or as intense as doing a ten-day retreat.

Mind Over Matter

Whether you are a beginner or an old-timer who has been meditating for years, there are many ways to start out or deepen your meditation journey.

One of the most profound concepts in this field is that of mindfulness, which lies at the heart of Buddhist meditation. Based on the idea that our current state of existence is limited by automaticity and unconsciousness, mindfulness cultivates a deeper connection with the present. It allows us to fully experience and appreciate each moment, without judgements or worries about the past or future that trap us in negative cycles of thought. Rather than a technique, mindfulness is a quality that can be gradually cultivated to infuse every waking moment and every activity with intention. Mindfulness meditation apps can help you practice this approach, focusing your mind on the present moment, observing when it is distracted and gently bringing it back.

In most forms of meditation, having a point of focus helps to tether the mind to the present, especially when you have a mind that tends to wander. The breath is an excellent place to start because it is always with us everywhere we go and because connecting to it has a profound impact on our bodies and minds. You might want to start simply by observing every breath you take or drawing attention to the sensations of the breath in your body. Gradually, you can begin to control your breath, counting the inhalations and exhalations, slowing down and drawing them out. Some people prefer other points of focus—an object such as a flame or a painting or even a chant of some sort.

If you're new to the practice, one of the best ways to begin is through guided meditation, where the voice of a teacher acts as an anchor for the mind. Starting out in complete silence and trying to empty the mind of thoughts can be more stressful than relaxing, whereas a teacher can break down the process for you, checking in with you and offering tips to gently draw the mind back to the point of focus. While meditation might appear to be a rather self-centred practice, it is part of a bigger approach that celebrates the oneness of life. In loving-kindness meditation, for example, you actively cultivate positivity for everyone and everything around you, starting with yourself and slowly radiating outwards to include family, friends, your tribe, nation and all living creatures of the world. One very simple way to start practicing this is to close your eyes and repeat the following or any other wish for wellbeing:

'May I be happy. May I be well. May I be safe. May I be peaceful and at ease.'

After you have done this for yourself, you can repeat the same for any number of people known and unknown to you.

While meditation is an ancient practice, dating back thousands of years, modern technology has managed to keep up and find ways to hack mindfulness. Going a step beyond guided meditation apps, there are now high-tech wearable devices that track brain waves during meditation and use neurofeedback to help train the mind for focus. The idea behind these devices is to observe, in real-time, how your brain is responding to different scenarios, whether stressful or relaxing. You then familiarize yourself with what each state feels like, learning how to avoid certain states and seek out others, especially during meditation. For example, the Muse headband, one of the more popular devices, uses electroencephalography (EEG) to translate your brain waves into the sounds of nature and the weather. Using neurofeedback, when your mind is calm and focused, you hear gentle, peaceful weather but if you are agitated or distracted, the weather turns stormy. This change is a signal to draw your attention back to the breath. As you do this more often, you begin to recognize the sensations associated with a still mind and can begin to train yourself to enter that state of calm.

We live in very exciting times. We are the inheritors of a rich legacy of ancients, who developed powerful insights and techniques to target the human mind over thousands of years. And now, we can experience these very techniques through the lens of modern technology, unravelling the biological underpinning and neural substrates that are involved in the functioning of the mind. The combined power of both is immensely transformative. Our entire existence is predicated on mental processes, while the body is just a vehicle to carry the mind and execute its wishes. Training and nurturing the mind is the most powerful thing one can do in the pursuit of a healthy life. Meditation is one of those bedrock habits that can not only make you feel better but also strengthen the mental prowess needed to practice other aspects of a healthy lifestyle. Hopefully, by now, you are convinced about the immense potential of any meditative practice and will seek out a technique or style to suit your taste and temperament. Take a deep breath and start living mindfully. No other way is worth it!

In Summary

Keep in Mind

1. Known as 'prana' in ancient Indian philosophy and 'qi' in Chinese traditions, breath has always been considered a centring life force, a theory validated by modern science.

2. Breathing happens both consciously, when we exert control over it, and unconsciously, involving the sympathetic and parasympathetic arms of the autonomic nervous system, making it a unique physiological process.

3. Breathing through the mouth and breathing too much—mouth breathing and over breathing—are the cause of many chronic health problems, as they leave the body in a state of constant stress.

4. A focus on breath during exercise and physical performance is important—nasal breathing during exercise can reduce exertion.

5. Different breathing techniques can help engage the diaphragm, boost relaxation and calm an anxious mind.

6. At the heart of meditation is cultivating the awareness to notice when the mind wanders or gets distracted and to gently draw it back to its point of focus.

7. Studies have found that meditation can alter brain function, making one less reactive and more resilient to stress, boosting wellbeing and health.

8. Meditation takes different forms, from focusing on the breath or an object to a chant or a feeling of compassion and loving kindness.

Take Action

1. Do a test to check if you're engaging the diaphragm when you breathe—while breathing deeply, place one palm on your abdomen and one on your chest. The hand on your chest should barely move, while the one on your abdomen should rise and fall.

2. Every time you notice yourself breathing through your mouth, make a conscious effort to close your mouth and switch to breathing through your nose. If you struggle to breathe through your nose, visit your doctor to check if you have allergies or other chronic ailments.

3. Avoid breathing too deep or too much as this can lead to hyperventilating and a state of stress. Slower breathing, with extended exhalations, can promote a feeling of calm.

4. Discuss breathing protocols during exercise with your trainer, understanding when to breathe through the nose and how long to hold inhalations and exhalations.

5. Guided meditation is the best way to begin a meditation practice, with a recorded voice or teacher checking in and giving you tips to draw your attention back when it wanders.

6. Good breathing practice is to slow down, extend exhalations and engage the diaphragm.

PART 3

TACKLING HEALTH GOALS

7

WEIGHT MANAGEMENT

Weight loss doesn't begin in the gym with a dumbbell; it starts in your head with a decision.—Toni Sorenson

It seems that the more progress we make, the fatter we become. The fatter we become, the greater the proliferation of weight loss solutions. The more we spend time and money on these solutions, the more weight we gain after temporarily losing some, eventually gaining some more for good measure before beginning the entire harrowing cycle afresh!

What's going on? With all the advancements in science and medicine, why is weight loss such a daunting problem? Why do we have such a propensity to gain weight at the first sign of prosperity? In this chapter we will take a close look at why weight gain is so easy, why weight loss is really hard, what science tells us about this and what you can do to truly achieve lasting weight loss.

I'd also like to clarify that when I talk about weight loss, I don't mean becoming skinny or achieving short-term aesthetic goals like a six-pack or a beach body. Weight loss here is about maintaining a healthy weight, because being overweight or obese is closely associated with a host of chronic health problems. This chapter is about weight loss for wellbeing rather than for aesthetics. In fact, fat is not fundamentally bad for us and, in addition to being a valuable source of energy, it is also responsible for managing several hormones in the body.

The Obesity Epidemic

People often point to the irony in the fact that until not long ago, we were fighting malnutrition and starvation, and yet, now the epidemic we face is that of obesity. According to the World Health Organization, obesity has tripled since 1975, with more than 1.9 billion overweight adults around the world, of which 650 million are obese. Most of the world's population now lives in countries where more people die from obesity and being overweight than from being underweight. In fact, things are now so dire that obesity is also affecting toddlers and young people. In 2019, thirty-eight million children under the age of five were obese. If this isn't an epidemic, I don't know what is.

Obesity is the excessive accumulation of fat that leads to various health complications from an unhealthy body weight. It is usually defined in terms of body mass index (BMI), a calculation of weight-for-height that is arrived at by dividing a person's weight in kilograms by the square of their height in metres. For adults, the WHO defines a BMI of 25 and above as overweight, and a BMI of 30 and above as obese. A BMI of 18.5–24.9 is healthy, and lower than 18.5 is underweight. Obesity is linked to numerous health problems, including cardiovascular disease, musculoskeletal disease and even some types of cancer. A good point to note is that while it is used in the definition of obesity, BMI is no longer considered an accurate measure of health or fitness. BMI only takes into account height and weight, and doesn't consider important elements like muscle mass, bone density and others. Instead, many people are now talking about body fat percentage. For example, a lean person with a low body fat percentage might have a high body weight because she has higher muscle mass, bone density or water in the body.

The most common understanding of obesity and weight gain is the 'calories in, calories out' theory which states that if we consume more calories than we expend through metabolic functions and physical activity, we will put on weight. It then stands to reason that if we consume fewer calories than we spend or if we spend more calories than we consume by exercising a lot, we will lose weight. Simple, right? Not quite, unfortunately. Many studies and researchers have recently discovered that this is a rather simplified view of things. If indeed it were simply a matter of calorie counting, how come all the awareness and implementation of diets and workouts, not to mention calorie counters and trackers, haven't had any impact on the rates of obesity?

Another idea that was often put forward to explain obesity was known as the 'thrifty gene' hypothesis, which claims that humans are evolutionarily predisposed to gain weight and store fat because of the scarcity of food our ancestors faced. And yet, morbid obesity is extremely rare in almost every species other than humans. Also, it's unlikely that humans would have benefitted from being overweight in the wild (imagine hunting, running from wild animals or navigating through rough terrain with all those extra kilograms piled on). In addition, societies that continue to follow traditional ways of life and diets have far lower rates of obesity than those that have switched over to the more modern or Western lifestyles.

In his fascinating book *The Obesity Code*, Dr Jason Fung argues that obesity is, in fact, a hormonal disorder related to insulin[1]. Insulin is the hormone responsible for regulating blood sugar levels, stimulating cells to take up glucose from the bloodstream to be used as fuel. Excess glucose is stored as glycogen in the liver and as fat in the body. Between meals or during periods of fasting, blood sugar and insulin levels drop, and the body begins to draw on the glycogen and fat stores for energy. However, when there aren't long enough gaps between meals, or when one's diet is too rich in refined carbohydrates and sugary foods, that cause the greatest spikes in blood sugar, the insulin levels remain consistently high. This throws off the fine balance of this system, leads to increased fat storage and can also disrupt the function of other hormones related to hunger and satiety.

Studies have found that in people of normal weight, insulin levels return to normal after a meal, while in overweight and obese people, the levels remain elevated for a longer period. Other studies have found that patients who are prescribed insulin to treat diabetes, gain weight. Dr Fung thus stipulates that increasing calories consumed and decreasing calories expended might not be the *cause* of obesity, but a *result* of this condition[2]. It's similar to what Gary Taubes writes in his book *Why We Get Fat*: 'We don't get fat because we overeat; we overeat because we're getting fat.'[3]

Therefore, diet is key, but not in the way that we thought. Instead of simply looking at calories, we need to look at *what* and *how* we eat. Diets high in refined carbohydrates, sugary food and drink, and low in whole, plant-based and fibre-rich food can lead to chronically high levels of insulin. In addition, constant snacking or grazing through the day, without long enough periods of fasting that allow insulin levels to drop, can also cause this chronic elevation. As a result of this, our cells can become insulin resistant, meaning that they no longer respond to the presence of the hormone to take up glucose from the blood. So, our blood sugar levels remain high, stimulating a further release of insulin. At the same time, our cells do not receive sufficient glucose and our bodies crave more food, further increasing blood glucose, insulin and, finally, weight.

Another cause for chronically high levels of insulin is an increase of the hormone cortisol in the body due to—you guessed it—stress. Cortisol regulates the fight-or-flight response to threat, and one of the outcomes is the increase in availability of glucose. Evolutionarily, this made sense as our ancestors probably needed the excess energy to run from a wild cat or chase down dinner. Modern stress, however, does not usually involve being chased by a predator (it's more likely to involve a stealthy, dangerous deadline) and is far more chronic. As a result, our blood sugar levels remain elevated over longer periods, stimulating the release of more insulin. In this way, stress plays an important role in the development of insulin resistance and resulting weight gain or obesity. Fortunately for you, if you go back to the chapter on meditation and sleep, you will find wonderful ways of dealing with stress in your life, and this could have a great impact on the way your body handles insulin and fat.

Why Weight Loss is Hard

While the 'calories in, calories out' theory seems to make sense on the surface, we also now know that weight loss is not *just* about consuming fewer calories than we expend or expending more calories than we consume by increasing physical activity. In fact, if it were as simple as that, it's unlikely that anyone would be overweight! Of course, taking care of one's nutrition and fitness are crucial ways of staying healthy and maintaining a healthy weight, but carrying around excess weight is not just a result of being greedy or lazy, as is often the assumption. In fact, being overweight is usually a symptom of an underlying issue, rather than a condition in itself. I have come to believe that this is often related to an imbalance of hormones, which is, in turn, generally a result of a diet high in refined carbohydrates, processed and sugary foods, as well as a sedentary, high stress lifestyle. The other element is related to our genes, which determine, to a large extent, how and where we put on weight, and how our bodies respond to nutrition and manage hormones like insulin.

After looking at studies about how weight gain happens and reading innumerable stories of weight loss struggles, I believe that there is something else at play. Over a lifetime of lifestyle choices related to what we eat, how often we eat, how active we are, what our stress levels are and so on, our bodies reach a kind of equilibrium weight. This could be 10–15 kg more than our ideal or desired weight. Barring the few people who might be severely obese, most people stay slightly overweight at a fixed point. This is a rather curious fact. If it was all about calories in and calories out, our weight would keep increasing indefinitely. This means that each of our bodies know what their equilibrium is based on our lifestyle and how our biological systems have been trained and maintain this weight with an almost religious fastidiousness. This is why, even when we manage to lose some weight, it doesn't take very long to bounce right back to our original weight, since crash diets don't overwrite the underlying biological mechanisms that are responsible for weight loss to begin with. To make meaningful and lasting weight loss happen, we need to rewire our biology, which takes time but is more effective. But perhaps more importantly, we also need to understand our equilibrium weight and be realistic about our weight goals.

One of the main reasons that losing weight is so hard, therefore, is that very few people have a sound understanding of why they are overweight in the first place. Instead, they follow one fad diet after another or sweat it out at random gym sessions, losing weight only to put it right back on again and realizing that the crash diet lifestyle is simply unsustainable. They end up living with a lack of self-esteem, believing that they must be as lazy and greedy as society has always said they were.

The other big problem is related to nutrition. We have talked about the bad reputation that fat has suffered for years, rather unfairly. Unfortunately, while much of the dialogue around fat is changing, many people still equate fat in the diet with becoming fat. As a result, many go the low-fat, high-carb route, which only messes with the mechanisms of the body that regulate insulin and blood sugar, actually leading to weight gain. It also doesn't help that the Western diet has flooded most supermarkets with the most highly refined versions of carbohydrates, as well as snacks and beverages that are filled with sugar. Most products that boast about being 'low-fat' forget to mention that they add on carbs and sugars to replace them.

Unfortunately, there is no quick fix when it comes to weight loss. It requires overhauling everything about your lifestyle, from the way you eat, drink and sleep to the way you work out and handle stress. And even after you make these changes, you will need patience to see the journey through, because the journey is a long one. And this is another reason why weight loss is so hard—most people simply give up when they don't see quick results. Imagine making really difficult changes in your life, such as giving up your favourite desserts and sugary drinks, sleeping at 9 p.m. every night, no matter how many social gatherings you might miss, or including a regular workout to your daily routine. And then imagine, that despite doing all of that, you don't see any difference at all on the weighing scale. That can be disheartening, and many people might lose all hope.

So, what can we do then? Do we throw up our hands in despair and blame it all on our bad genes? An innate tendency to put on weight is beyond anyone's control. However, the way we live our lives determines whether this tendency gets turned on or not. Making a simple choice to avoid processed foods, refined carbs and sweetened and sugary drinks and products is one step that will take you a long way. Considering stress also plays a role in weight gain, learning to manage your response to stressors can also help manage your weight. Quality of sleep, as we saw in an earlier chapter, also has a significant impact on weight, by affecting levels of the hunger hormone ghrelin and the satiety hormone leptin. Focusing on all of these, while also developing a fitness habit, can help you manage weight, even if your genes might be working against you.

CRASH DIETS

A crash diet is one in which users severely restrict caloric intake over a short period of time to lose weight very quickly. The exact method might vary—from doing a lemon juice cleanse to eating nothing but cabbage soup for a week—but the ultimate goal remains the same: shedding weight quickly. However, most crash diets quite literally crash (pardon the terrible pun) when any weight that is lost is put back on almost as quickly—sometimes with even more weight as a bonus. Most people go on crash diets for very specific purposes—to fit into an outfit, to look great on a beach vacation or for a big event. While there's nothing wrong with having an aesthetic ideal or a goal in mind, a crash diet is rarely a sustainable method of weight loss in the long term. In fact, not only do people often end up putting on more weight than they lost, but they might also end up with various health problems they didn't have before going on the diet.

There's one recurring lesson that you might have noticed cropping up throughout this book . . . there are no shortcuts! And crash diets are shortcuts that look like they're working in the short-term but end up wreaking havoc after you have shown off your beach body on that holiday or squeezed into your oldest suit or dress for a destination wedding. While you might see the scale shifting downwards in the aftermath of the diet, this can often be the result of losing lean muscle mass and water. Severely restricting calorie intake can also lead to feelings of intense hunger and an unhealthy obsession with food.

In fact, theories say that when you reduce the number of calories that you feed the body, the body adapts by reducing its energy expenditure. This reduces resting metabolic rate and thermogenesis to save energy, as the body thinks it is preparing for starvation. In response to this, it actually stores fat and burns lean muscle, making you feel sluggish and tired. By the third day of a crash diet, hormonal function is affected. This results in extreme mood swings and intense cravings for food. And within a week, up to 50 per cent of weight loss might be from the loss of lean muscle, while the body will start missing key nutrients. By the end of the diet, or a month, you feel so deprived that you probably go on a binge of all your favourite unhealthy goodies. By this point, your body goes into fat storage overdrive to replenish its stores, having just experienced what it considered a period of starvation. And if you thought it couldn't get any worse, this entire experience can have a profound effect on body positivity and self-esteem, leaving one feeling worthless and miserable.

Fat Metabolism

Fat has gone from being considered a masterful stroke of evolution that allowed our ancestors to store energy during seasons of abundance for times of scarcity, to a symbol of wealth, to a reviled nutrient associated with obesity and heart disease. It might be hard to imagine, but there was a time in the late nineteenth and early twentieth centuries when there were clubs celebrating corpulence as a sign of prosperity. One of the sayings of one such group was: 'A fat bank account tends to make a fat man.' Some clubs had weigh-ins to find the member who weighed the most, and many involved eating a great deal of food at their meetings, but all of them considered being fat a matter of pride.[4] Fast forward to a mere few decades later, and suddenly popular culture was filled with stick-thin models, and before we knew it, being fat was equated with being lazy, sloth-like and gluttonous. Only recently have we begun to truly understand the nature of fat and its relationship with our health.

Fat plays a role in moderating the body's stores of energy, in the development and function of the brain, as well as in nutrient absorption. In fact, fat is now defined as an organ[5], and considered a dynamic element involved in the body's health.

From our food, some dietary fat is stored directly in our fat tissues as fatty acids, while the rest is processed by the liver along with carbohydrates, sugars and proteins, and converted into fat for storage. The fat molecules produced in the liver are transported through the bloodstream to be deposited in the cells of the body, particularly in our fat cells. Fat molecules are chains of carbon atoms in sets of three that make triglycerides, which are long and malleable, making them easy to pack tightly into the body's fat cells. Fat is a super dense source of energy, as its molecules repel water and can be packed in together very tightly—in fact, 40,000 calories of fat weighs under 5 kg! When the body has used up available glucose in the blood and also burned through its store of glycogen in the liver, it begins to metabolize fats.

The thing about fat, like the thing about many aspects of life, is that it can be good and bad. Subcutaneous fat is the fat that is more visible, just under the skin, while visceral fat is the kind that forms between and around the body's organs. Visceral fat can be more dangerous than subcutaneous, because it secretes more hormones and promotes inflammation. Therefore, it is more positively associated with insulin resistance, diabetes, as well as heart disease and high cholesterol. One of the hormones that helps subcutaneous fat play its role in good health is adiponectin, which orchestrates the insulin response, drawing glucose and fat out of the bloodstream. By removing excess fats from circulation, subcutaneous fat removes a precursor for diabetes. The hormone adiponectin helps to understand why all obese people are not unhealthy or suffer from type 2 diabetes—they have higher levels of good fat, which actually helps keep them stay healthy. Exercise helps balance good fat and bad fat by increasing the levels of adiponectin and reducing the amount of visceral fat.

HEALTH HACK #19: Kombucha

Kombucha is an ancient fermented drink that originated in northeast China in 200 B.C., made using black or green tea and a symbiotic culture of bacteria and yeast. Thanks to its probiotic effects, kombucha is excellent for digestive health, as well as immunity.

Sugar & Insulin

Being overweight or obese is so often and so closely linked to being diabetic, that the term diabesity is one that is now often used. Studies have found that, although obesity is defined as having a BMI of 25 or over, women with a BMI of 23–23.9 are 360 per cent more likely to develop diabetes than those with a BMI of 22 or less. In addition, researchers have found that a weight gain of 5–7.9 kg increases the risk for type 2 diabetes by 90 per cent, while a weight gain of eight to 10.9 kg increases that risk by 270 per cent! The risk for diabetes can, conversely, be reduced by up to 50 per cent by losing weight. Therefore, while talking about weight loss, it's absolutely vital to acknowledge the intricate relationship between diet, insulin, blood sugar and weight gain.

It's now well understood that carbohydrates in the diet break down into glucose when digested. However, different types of carbohydrates have different effects on blood glucose levels, and this is measured by something known as the glycaemic index. Foods rich in sugar and refined carbohydrates have the highest glycaemic index, as they raise the blood glucose levels significantly and quickly. Among the worst of the sugars are sucrose or table sugar, and high-fructose corn syrup (HFCS). The biggest problem with sweeteners like HFCS is that they contain a combination of fructose and glucose, which are both metabolized differently. While glucose directly enters circulation and raises blood sugar levels, fructose is processed in the liver. Thus, while it doesn't immediately impact blood sugar and insulin levels, it has a longer-term negative effect, contributing to the development of insulin resistance and weight gain.

If you suspect your weight gain might be related to your body's insulin mechanism, it might be a good idea to regularly check your blood sugar levels. A diet that is rich in fibre, with lots of fruit, vegetables, legumes, lentils and other low glycaemic foods, can also help to keep blood sugar levels in check.

A Diet Plan for Weight Loss

When we say that the answer to weight loss doesn't lie in cutting calories, this doesn't mean we can eat anything we want, any time we want it. A diet plan for weight loss is more about eating patterns and food habits, rather than merely the number of calories and the kinds of calories on your plate. Here are some simple rules of thumb to follow if you want to eat healthy and shed some extra kilograms:

1. Build your meals around plant-based sources of food which are not calorie-dense but are high in fibre, antioxidants and flavonoids, among other good stuff. If you eat meat and dairy, try to make sure at least 70–80 per cent of your calories come from plants.

2. Planning meals that are balanced and nutritious is super important because, if you simply reduce calories, you might end up feeling constantly hungry. If your breakfast is carb-heavy, you're probably not going to feel satiated very long, leading to constant snacking or overeating through the rest of the day.

3. Low protein intake might actually cause sugar cravings, so cutting out too much protein in an effort to lose weight could be counterintuitive.

4. A simple way of ensuring truly balanced meals that leave you feeling full is to add good fats like ghee, nuts and coconut to your breakfasts and other meals, which will cut down your food cravings and ensure better weight management in the long term.

5. Incorporating some form of fasting in your day is a good idea—you could start by giving yourself a 'no seconds' rule or skip dinner a few times a week and see how you feel.

6. Snacking is more often related to habit and easy accessibility
    of deliciously salty and crunchy food items than actual hunger
    pangs. So, try to clear out that snack cupboard, and if you
    really need a bite of something with your afternoon tea, try
    sticks of carrot and cucumber, apple with peanut butter, or a
    handful of nuts instead.
7. Women with PCOS often struggle with managing their weight,
    and it is important to avoid inflammatory foods, as well as meat
    injected with antibiotics. The gut microbiome also undergoes
    changes during PMS, leading to food cravings. It is important
    to focus on low-glycaemic foods like root vegetables and
    tubers, as well as natural and supplemental forms of vitamin E
    to reduce cravings and excess calorie consumption.
8. For most of us, our weight during the day may fluctuate by as
    much as 2–3 kg, depending on the time of day, bowel movements
    and water intake. While it may be useful to weigh in every week
    or fortnight, observing your weight on a monthly basis will offer
    a more realistic picture of where you are headed.
9. Most importantly, as you design your diet plan, remember that
    it must be sustainable. Don't try anything too drastic, because it
    won't last, and it might leave you feeling fatigued and constantly
    hungry. If you have any chronic illnesses, it's best to work closely
    with a doctor or nutritionist to plan your meals.

A FITNESS PLAN FOR WEIGHT LOSS

Just as a diet plan needs to be something you can sustain over the
long run without feeling miserable, a fitness plan for weight loss
also needs to be practical with attainable goals. The good news
here is that any form of physical activity is good for you and burns
calories. Below are a few tips and tricks for an effective fitness plan,
if weight loss is your goal:

1. Walking is the best place to start—it's easy, accessible and can be done anywhere. If you have a fitness tracker, a good place to start is to get 10,000 steps a day. Not only is walking one of the best forms of exercise for weight loss, it also increases your energy levels and provides you with a much needed break from your desk and screens.

2. Cardio workouts of all kinds, from running to Zumba, are effective ways to burn calories while having fun. The thing to keep in mind is that you are likely to feel extra hungry after, so have a meal with complex carbs about two hours before your workout or a fruit about 30–45 minutes before.

3. After any intense exercise, it's a good idea to have a protein-rich snack or supplement to prevent fatigue, as well as to ensure you don't overeat at your next meal. Proteins provide the building blocks to repair wear and tear in the body and leave you feeling satiated longer.

4. HIIT is an excellent form of exercise that can also be done in a relatively short period of time. Some experts say that metabolism remains high after an HIIT workout, giving you the 'afterburn' effect.

5. Despite its association with bulking up, weight training is also a good way to lose weight because muscle burns more calories at rest than most other tissues. Resting metabolism also increases straight after a weight training session, and this effect lasts longer than after a cardio workout.

6. Working closely with a trainer and keeping your goals realistic can help you create a workout plan that you can effectively sustain.

In Summary

Keep in Mind

1. Obesity, or the unhealthy accumulation of fat, is an epidemic across the world, closely linked to the development of lifestyle diseases.
2. While people have commonly assumed obesity to be a result of laziness and greed, recent research shows it could be a hormonal disorder related to insulin.
3. Weight loss is not just about eating less and exercising more; it requires an understanding of our individual biology and overhauling our lifestyle and habits.
4. Our bodies seem to have an equilibrium weight, the result of genetics and accumulated lifestyle choices, which it bounces back to despite efforts to lose more.
5. Crash diets require severe restriction of calories, and given that this is not sustainable, they often result in bouncing right back to the original weight or even gaining more.
6. Despite its bad reputation, fat is now being recognized as an incredibly important aspect of a healthy body and a crucial source of energy.
7. Being overweight drastically increases the risk of diabetes. Sugary foods and refined carbohydrates interfere with the system of insulin and blood sugar regulation.

Take Action

1. Figure out what your equilibrium or set point weight is— this is likely to be the weight that you have been for most of your adult life, despite lifestyle or other changes. Your goal

weight should be close to this point in order to be realistic and achievable.

2. If you find yourself either gaining or losing weight, despite taking steps to do the opposite, it might be a good idea to speak to your doctor and take a hormone test.

3. A plant-based diet, a system of intermittent fasting, restricting yourself to one serving per meal, or even occasionally skipping a meal are good ways of losing weight sustainably.

4. Any kind of workout from walking and running to Zumba, HIIT and weightlifting are good ways of exercising to lose weight—as long as your exercise plan is sustainable.

8

KEEPING DISEASE AT BAY

No doctor has ever healed anyone of anything in the history of the world, The human immune system heals and that's the only thing that heals.—Bob Wright

I would like to be able to tell you that I've been healthy throughout my life, but the truth is that there was a time I really struggled to stay well. In my twenties and thirties, I had the tendency to fall sick every six months to one year. Assuming this was normal, I never really paid much attention to it. I ended up taking several courses of antibiotics during this period—probably far too many for my gut health. Things hit rock bottom when I moved back to India in 2007. I went from falling sick once or twice a year to feeling unwell every single month. I visited several doctors and took various courses of medications until I finally consulted an expert. Looking at my history, he grew worried—so worried, in fact, that he asked me to do an HIV test. Fortunately, the result was negative, and it seemed like my immunity was just really low.

This was around the time that I had just moved back to India after a decade in the US. The change in environment, combined with the stress of running an early stage start-up, a poor diet and a lack of exercise, are probably what led to my state of dangerously compromised immunity. This experience alarmed me enough to start taking my health and my immune system more seriously. I started with just trying to get the basics right—getting more sleep, starting on a consistent fitness routine and paying more attention to the food I ate. I gradually began to see the impact of a healthier lifestyle on my immunity.

These days, I have taken things to the next level. Having done a lot of reading on the latest science of immunity and recovery, I have started experimenting with some of the more cutting-edge technologies, alongside traditional remedies and therapies. Every morning, I drink an immunity-boosting turmeric-based drink and on weekends, when I have more time, I take steam and ice baths. In fact, I recently got a Morozko Forge—an ice bath machine that makes its own ice-cold water and in which I can set my preferred temperature to get the most benefits. I also take various supplements that are known for their benefits to the immune system.

With all the changes I have made to my lifestyle, from sleep and fitness to incorporating supplements and recovery protocols in my regime, I have found a way to stay healthier. I now hardly ever fall sick. In fact, I seem to have managed to dodge the virus during the pandemic, and while I might have just got lucky, I do think that my boosted immunity played a role too. My work required me to travel almost every week between the second and third waves, but fortunately, my immunity managed to keep any viral infection at bay. While we each have our own health goals— managing or preventing lifestyle diseases, perhaps, or losing or gaining weight—immunity forms an important foundation to achieve these. In this chapter, we will look at immunity and lifestyle diseases in some detail to understand the different health journeys that we will all take at some point in our lives.

* * *

The 1976 film, *The Boy in the Plastic Bubble*, starring John Travolta, featured a boy with immune deficiencies that forced him to live his entire life inside a completely sterile environment. This and the 2001 film, *Bubble Boy*, were both loosely based on the lives of two young boys in America—Ted DeVita who had aplastic anaemia, meaning his body could not produce enough blood cells including immune cells, and David Vetter, who suffered severe combined immunodeficiency (SCID). Both were confined to small, sterile settings, where their interactions with the world around them was very limited. We often take our immunity for granted, but these stories illustrate just how difficult—and even impossible—it would be to live without these beautifully evolved systems of defence, which allow us to experience and enjoy all that the world has to offer.

The COVID-19 pandemic that raged across the globe in 2020 and 2021, wreaking unimaginable havoc and bringing the world to a standstill, was a powerful reminder that no matter how advanced we might be as a species, we are still incredibly vulnerable to disease. It awakened memories and stories of illnesses that have changed the course of human history, politics and society. The Roman Empire, one of the most powerful of the ancient world, was decimated by the Antonine Plague of 165–180 AD, now believed to be a smallpox epidemic. Then, its population was ravaged by the Plague of Justinian in 541 AD. These terrible illnesses, that wiped out a significant number of lives, contributed to the decline and eventual downfall of the great empire. In the past, humans sought divine intervention, praying to the gods and goddesses for protection. In fact, statues of South Asia's first 'epidemic' goddess, Hariti, date back to the time of the Antonine Plague, indicating that she might have been worshipped as a deity that shielded her people from smallpox.

While people might still find solace in prayer and worship, we, fortunately, now have something else on our side when it comes to facing illness—and that is science. The coronavirus disease brought the field of immunity into the spotlight, making it front page news, and rightly so. While tens of millions are exposed to the deadly virus, it became apparent that most developed only mild symptoms, if any, while a small percentage progressed to more advanced stages of the disease. This is, perhaps, one of the most visible demonstrations of the role immunity plays in our lives and health—making us more susceptible to life-threatening diseases when it is weak but keeping us alive when it is at its strongest. In addition, the record breaking speed with which the vaccines were developed is testament to just how far the science of immunity has come.

Immunity is not just important in the context of pandemics, but also in our day to day lives. Being laid low by a flu or any kind of illness can take a toll on our productivity at work, our fitness routines and our health in the long-term. An understanding of the intricacies of the immune system and ways to shore it up can help us build long-lasting good health, better resilience to disease and save precious time otherwise lost to ill health. If you don't understand the intricacies of the immune system and find ways to shore it up, you're likely to lose precious time to ill health and suffer the consequences for a long time. Immunity is a foundational pillar for long-lasting good health—ensuring that everything else, from a healthy diet to a fit body, becomes more sustainable.

WHAT IS IMMUNITY

Immunity has been defined as 'the global ability of the host to resist the predation of microbes that would otherwise destroy it'.[1] As we go about our daily lives, we are exposed constantly to the external world, through the air we breathe, the food we eat, the water we drink and the numerous objects and surfaces we come into contact with. If not for our immune system, we would be knocked down by every microscopic organism we happened to encounter, constantly falling sick. Immunity, therefore, is a state of resistance to disease or infection.

The immune system is one of the most ancient organ systems that predates the evolution of the human species. Scientists have discovered that bacteria, which were the first cellular organisms to appear on earth, developed an advanced immune response, allowing them to create memories of specific threats to them, so they could be neutralized the next time they were encountered.

One of the core ideas on which the study of immunology is based is that our immune system helps us to distinguish between the 'self' and 'non-self': the ability to recognize that which belongs to and is part of the body and that which is a foreign 'invader' posing a threat. This almost existential consciousness is what allows the intricate immune system to mount the most effective defence against the threat. The complexity of human immunity is evident in the fact that the cells of our bodies seem to learn and remember from every attack, to protect us better from similar invaders in the future.

The immune system doesn't have an easy time of it, however. Not only does it need to be constantly on the lookout for bad guys by monitoring everything we eat, breathe or otherwise come into contact with, but it also needs to allow cell growth for repair while keeping an eye out for damaged or mutated cells. It is when these processes are disrupted that people end up with autoimmune disorders, in which the system turns on itself, or with cancers, in which bad cells are allowed to proliferate. The cells of our immune system are like security guards that work 24X7, having to constantly look out for possible threats. They are further divided into various kinds of special forces, for different types of attack.

Our immunity functions in an elegant two-system response format, known as the innate and the adaptive immune systems. These two systems work together in precise and beautiful harmony to protect us from various pathogens.

The innate immune system is the first line of defence in the body, that is activated immediately when disease-causing bacteria or viruses enter the body. It comprises physical barriers, such as the skin and mucous membranes, chemical barriers, such as sweat, saliva or digestive enzymes, and biological barriers, including the good bacteria that live in our gut and other parts of the body.

Lymphocytes, monocytes, basophils, neutrophils and eosinophils are the five types of white blood cells that drive the immune system, and lymphocytes are kind of the star players. There are two types of lymphocytes—B-cells that mature in the bone marrow and T-cells that are trained in the thymus. Killer T-cells destroy infected cells, helper T-cells support other immune cells and memory T-cells store memories of earlier infections so they can launch a speedy attack if the same foreign body invades again. The latter method is known as adaptive immunity, and a good example is chicken pox—once you've had it, the memory T-cells are so good at their job that they can protect you from getting it again. B-cells produce proteins known as antibodies which can destroy invading pathogens.

One of the many incredible things about our immune system is that it seems to be very well equipped to handle a variety of pathogens, some that we may or may not even encounter in our entire lifetimes. When we travel to foreign countries, eat new types of food, drink water from unfamiliar sources, we come into contact with new bacteria that have the potential to harm us. And yet, it seems that our bodies possess the antibodies to respond to the antigens expressed by these entirely foreign pathogens.

Inflammation is the body's response to infection, experienced as swelling, heat, pain and redness at the site of infection or injury. This is the result of blood vessels dilating to bring more white blood cells to the region—which can enter the injured tissues and get to work. White blood cells release chemicals known as cytokines that lead to the actual symptoms of illness, such as fever, discomfort or pain.

This is a very simple introduction to what is an extremely complex system. The various elements we've discussed come together in exquisite harmony, through an incredibly intricate system of communication and signalling, to keep us in the best of health. The precision of this balance is what gives us immunity and therefore, keeps us alive.

HEALTH HACK #20: MedWand

Thanks to the COVID-19 pandemic, many of us began to consult our doctors online for health questions. While video and audio technology are familiar to all of us, devices like the MedWand are truly transforming telemedicine. The MedWand can measure and record the key vitals in real-time while a doctor is consulting with a patient via video conferencing. With technology like this, we might not need to visit a clinic or a hospital to consult a doctor ever again.

WHY DO WE FALL SICK?

The simple answer to the question about why we fall sick is that disease-causing microorganisms or pathogens, including bacteria, viruses and parasites, enter our bodies and infect our cells. This can happen when we are exposed to other sick people, for example, or when we eat or drink something that has gone bad. These pathogens are very good at crossing the body's barriers, the skin or the gut, for example, and at evading the body's defences, by multiplying and mutating at alarming rates. It can all get pretty nasty, but fortunately for us, our body has a natural system of defence in the form of immunity.

The symptoms of sickness, such as a fever, a leaky nose, a bad stomach or a rash, are actually signs that our immune system is at work, trying to eliminate or digest the infected cells. This happens through the generalized mechanisms and physical barriers of the innate immune system as it goes into high gear. Inflammation is the body's way of securing the point of attack, by sending its foot soldiers or immune cells to the defence. The swelling around an injury or a stuffy nose, therefore, are also signs that the system is in order and the healing process has begun.

Raising temperature helps the body fight infection, by directly affecting pathogens—for example, the rate of replication in viruses decreases by 200 times at temperatures of 104 degrees Fahrenheit—and by boosting immune system activity, such as increasing the number of immune cells entering the bloodstream. Interestingly, cold-blooded animals are not like warm-blooded ones, in that, they cannot alter their body temperature through altered metabolic activity. Instead, however, some of them, like iguanas and tuna fish, are able to change their body temperature by seeking out warmer environments when they experience infection, a phenomenon known as 'heat seeking' behaviour. Studies have also found that medicines known to treat fevers in warm-blooded creatures can reduce this heat seeking behaviour in cold-blooded animals. And just in case that isn't fascinating enough, there are even certain plants that experience fevers—raising temperature to fight fungal infections.

Many pathogens have evolved very sophisticated mechanisms to evade our body's immune system. For example, the salmonella-causing bacteria develop a capsule-like shell to protect itself, while some staphylococcus bacteria mimic human cells so that our immune system doesn't recognize them as a foreign invader.

GONE BATTY

Apart from its vampiric associations, few of us would consider the bat as anything other than an innocuous if slightly mysterious creature of the night. However, with the discovery that bats were the source of the Nipah, SARS and Ebola outbreaks, and might have also caused the COVID-19 pandemic, the way we view this mammal is changing. Recent studies have found that bats might be a 'reservoir species' thanks to their unique immune systems. For one, bats are constantly 'exercising', putting them in a fever state that might prevent them from falling ill when infected by a virus. In addition, bats were found to have high levels of interferons, immune substances that help eliminate viruses, and lower levels of inflammatory cytokines. Both allow them to carry viruses without falling victim to symptoms. Finally, environmental factors—like drought, increasing temperatures and loss of habitat—lead to bats migrating, taking the viruses with them, from where they spread to human communities.

We are particularly susceptible to falling sick when our defences are weakened, and this can happen because of chronic stress, sleep deprivation and even poor nutrition and fitness. Studies have found that people who are chronically stressed are at greater risk for viral infections, while their wounds take longer to heal and their response to vaccines diminishes. Increased levels of cortisol in response to stress dampens the immune response and reduces the immune system's efficiency.

Sleep and immunity are intimately connected as well, with sleep deprivation having similar effects to stress. People who are chronically sleep-deprived tend to have a poor response to vaccines. This could mean that a fatigued immune system is not able to learn a new immune response. In addition, a lack of sleep leads to changes in at least ten interleukins, types of cytokines that regulate the immune response. What's interesting is that a healthy immune system, in turn, can improve sleep by producing cytokines, some of which promote sleep. This relationship also makes sense if you think about how fatigued and sleepy you feel when you're sick—this is your immune system telling you to rest and leave more resources available to fight infection. So, in fact, it's not the virus that's making you feel lethargic and exhausted, but substances in the body such as interferon, the signalling proteins released by cytokines.

Given that part of our immune system resides in our gut, our diet plays an important role in our defences. One study, in fact, found that when certain bacteria are not present in our gut, the immune system cannot produce T-cells. In addition, it has been discovered that gut bacteria actually send signals that stimulate the development of immune cells.

Exercise and immunity seem to have a love–hate relationship. Moderate intensity exercise is associated with better immune health and anti-inflammatory effects. However, prolonged periods of intense exercise without adequate recovery can lead to a depressed immune system and an onslaught of infections. This might be why athletes, after training and game season, often fall victim to the flu and other illnesses. A 2019 review of exercise immunology, as this field of study is called, discovered that moderate exercise improved the circulation of immune cells in the body, enhancing the levels and activity of certain cells, including natural killer cells.

Conversely, the physiological and psychological stress brought on by intense exercise over prolonged periods are found to lead to immune cell dysfunction and inflammation.

THE HYGIENE HYPOTHESIS, ALLERGIES & OVERREACTIONS

While better and more hygienic living conditions mean that we no longer suffer or die from everyday infections, there is a theory that this, in fact, presents a problem. According to the 'hygiene hypothesis', living in extremely clean and sterile environments means that we miss out on essential exposure to germs that would teach our immune systems when and how to launch a defence against pathogens. While we have the same immune systems that our ancestors did, we have drastically changed and sterilized the spaces we inhabit—purifying the water we drink and the air we breathe, using pesticides to kill organisms on the crops we eat and over sanitizing our homes. As a result, our immune system begins to overreact to harmless things like dust mites or pollen, developing allergies, chronic immune attacks, inflammation and asthma.

One example of this comes from the Amish and Hutterites, who belong to communal ethno-religious groups that have similar roots and live in what they call 'intentional communities' in the United States. Farmers from both communities share many genetic, social and cultural traits, except for the fact that the Amish refuse to use technology, while the Hutterites have embraced it. As a result, Amish children grow up spending far more time outdoors, rather than on their iPads, and are constantly in contact with their livestock. This is credited for their lower rates of asthma compared to Hutterite children, thanks to the hygiene hypothesis. Other studies have found that children who grow up with pets or with older siblings are less susceptible to allergies and autoimmune conditions, as a result of increased exposure to germs from a young age.

Histamines are chemicals produced by the immune system to get rid of anything that is bothering it. When the trigger is an allergen—usually something harmless like dust or pollen—histamines go into overdrive, trying its best to get rid of what it sees as a major threat. The immune system sets off this chain reaction, causing inflammation at the point of entry—for example, your nose—where histamines cause the production of more mucus, leading to a runny nose, sneezing, itchy eyes and other symptoms of an allergy. This is one example of the immune system overreacting. Another is something that unfortunately became more common in some cases of severe COVID-19 infection, spotlighting the intricate balance maintained by our immune system. In certain cases, due to infection, disease, autoimmune conditions or certain therapies, the body releases too many cytokines into the blood. This flood of cytokines known as a cytokine storm, which are a part of our normal immune response, can lead to hyperinflammation, causing high fevers and fatigue, leading, in certain extreme cases, to multiorgan failure.

Boosting Immunity

One can visualize the immune system as a fortification designed to keep us safe from invading pathogens, but the strength of this shield can be depleted due to a poor lifestyle, leaving it full of holes and vulnerabilities. But it doesn't have to be that way. Our immune system responds wonderfully to our lifestyle and, with careful choices, we can considerably boost its strength, making us less susceptible to illness, improving the quality of life and also possibly helping us live longer!

Let's start with the fundamentals. Most of the things that are part of an overall healthy lifestyle play an important role in boosting immunity as well. The following are some of the most basic elements:

- Getting seven to nine hours of sleep a night will give your body the opportunity it needs to replenish depleted immune cells and build up its defence.
- A diet rich in fruit and veggies will give you the vitamins and minerals that your immunity needs to function at its best.
- Mindfulness practices, nature walks and other relaxing activities can fend off the stress that depletes our immunity.
- Regular, moderate exercise can recharge and regenerate the immune system. One needs to be careful though, as very strenuous exercise can reduce immunity and needs to be compensated with significantly increased rest periods.
- Regular health checkups and adequate supplements when required can address immunity issues related to specific deficiencies.

Good nutrition supports the healthy functioning of the immune system, while fuelling the great energy demand placed on the body when it is fighting infection. Several vitamins and micronutrients, including vitamins A, C and D, zinc and specific amino acids, that we get from our diet increase the effectiveness of immune function. Since so much of our immune system resides in the gut, eating a healthy diet high in whole, natural, plant-based foods and foods that support a balanced gut microbiome can improve your immunity.

Addressing stress and mental health through interventions like meditation can be good for our immune system too. In fact, traditional Chinese medicine has viewed cancer as a result of emotional distress as much as physiological. Research has also discovered a connection between depression and a weakened immune response. These connections stem from the fact that our gut microbiota is not only responsible for digestion, but is also intimately involved in both our mood, as well as our immune systems.

One of the most illustrative examples of how stress affects immunity is in the case of the herpes virus. Among the most common virus families, the herpes virus has double-stranded DNA, similar to the human DNA, which can be a bit confusing for the immune system. In addition, the herpes virus often lies dormant in the body, where the immune cells keep an eye on it without attacking it. However, when we undergo any kind of stress, the virus seems to sense the weakness, taking advantage of the opening to attack.

They say that laughter is the best medicine, and surprisingly, there are some studies that have looked into the link between humour and immunity. It is assumed that laughter and funny situations help combat the ill effects of stress, but some research has actually found an increase in salivary IgA, the main antibody in saliva and mucus, after exposure to a humorous stimulus.[2] The fact is, though, that stress has a powerful negative impact on our immune systems, and any efforts to better manage stress can help.

To boost your immunity, try and get your diet, fitness and sleep routines back on track, while trying to control stress through mindful healing practices. A well-equipped immune system can help form the basis of a healthy lifestyle.

HEALTH HACK #21: Cupping

Several ancient traditional healing systems around the world used cupping—the use of cups placed on the body using heat or suction. Research into this form of therapy is underway, but it is used in pain relief, recovery in athletes, as well as to treat skin diseases and improve immune function.

IMMUNITY HACKS

Beyond caring for your immune system by making better long-term health choices, there are also some great hacks and secrets that many high performers have discovered and now swear by.

One of the most unexpected might be to eat less, or even practice some light fasting, during flu season. This might sound counterintuitive, because we've often been told to eat a substantial amount of food to 'boost' our recovery. However, the only really substantial thing in this situation is the amount of energy the body uses for digestion, thus diverting fuel required by the immune system to shore itself up. Eating light or skipping meals, avoiding sugar and heavy, starchy food could all help your immune system fight back. This mild starvation mode triggers survival circuits, which is why Ayurveda often treats illness by restricting the number of meals to avoid taxing the body.

We have all heard about how the sun's harmful UV radiation can suppress the immune system, but more recent research has said that some exposure to sunlight might actually boost immunity, by increasing vitamin D levels and activating T-cells. The answer lies in limiting your exposure to the sun to under thirty minutes in the mornings, to make sure you can tap into its healing powers without risking its adverse effects.

Ben Greenfield has a whole list of hacks when it comes to developing his 'unstoppable' immunity. One, that might sound rather absurd, involves Ben jumping on a trampoline! He does this, an activity known as rebounding, or uses a vibration platform, in order to increase lymph flow in the body, enhancing drainage and filtration within the lymphatic system, which plays a key role in immunity. A visit to a chiropractor, sweating profusely in a sauna, dry skin brushing and massages can all have similar effects to rebounding and vibration. Greenfield also swears by bone broth, fermented foods, including homemade yoghurt, which used to be a staple of most Indian homes, as well as echinacea and a herbal concoction known as Thieves Oil containing essential oils like eucalyptus, cinnamon and lemon.

While the antioxidant effects of vitamin C are well known, many of us also pop vitamin C pills to treat the common cold. Studies have shown that supplementing with vitamin C doesn't have much of an effect on a cold, although supplementing with this vitamin before or at the onset of a cold might be beneficial. However, the best sources for vitamin C are natural—citrus fruits like oranges, grapefruit and lemon, non-citrus fruits like papaya and strawberry, as well as green leafy vegetables and cruciferous vegetables like cauliflower. Many biohackers and high performers, however, take things a bit further by getting a high-dose injection of vitamin C every few months. High doses cannot be taken orally, as they can cause an upset stomach.

Zinc might be one of the best ways in which to hack your immunity. Not only does this micronutrient—found in meat, cheese and seafood—have antioxidant and anti-inflammatory properties, it is also a component of many, many proteins and enzymes that are essential for immunity. Zinc works best when taken at the onset of symptoms of a cold or flu, as it interferes with the replication of a virus. Interestingly, zinc also helps address the loss of taste and smell that often accompany a cold— symptoms that are linked to COVID-19 as well. It's also most effective in the form of ionic zinc, as lozenges, which slowly release the micronutrient into the nasal and throat passages to nip sickness in the bud.

VACCINES & ANTIBIOTICS

In his book, *The Elegant Defense: The Extraordinary New Science of the Immune System*, Matt Richtel calls vaccines the 'boot camp for the immune system'[3] because they are literally aimed at training the body's T-cells and B-cells. A vaccine contains an agent that resembles a pathogen or contains the actual weakened or dead microorganism or its protein, equipping our adaptive immune system to respond faster and more effectively to specific diseases. However, a vaccine has to be perfectly developed to be effective enough to stimulate the immune response, but not so powerful that it causes harm. In fact, the history of the vaccine features rather horrific chapters, including one in which a test polio vaccine left children paralysed. Even after Jonas Salk developed an effective polio vaccine, one batch that was improperly produced led to paralysis and even death in the children it was administered to. Fortunately, polio was eventually eradicated with the right vaccine. All of this just goes to show the delicate balance and beautiful complexity of the human immune system.

Antibiotics are medicines that inhibit the growth of or destroy harmful bacteria in the human body. They take advantage of certain differences between human and bacterial cells, one of which is a wall that bacterial cells have, which humans do not. In some cases, antibiotics inhibit the growth of this wall within the human host. The discovery of the first antibiotic is relatively well known now. The Scotsman, Dr Alexander Fleming, had a petri dish filled with strep bacteria, his subject of study. One day, he observed that a part of the dish suddenly no longer had this lethal bacteria. On further study, Fleming realized that mould growing in the dish seemed to be killing the bacteria. This mould went on to win Fleming a Nobel Prize, when he turned it into the medicine we now know as penicillin.

A key difference between a vaccine and an antibiotic is that the vaccine is boosting our inborn immune response, while antibiotics are essentially interfering with the natural process. As a result, antibiotics must be treated with a fair amount of wariness and not as pills you can pop at the first signs of a stomach or throat infection. If you've read the section on the gut, you will know that our body is host to innumerable friendly and harmless bacteria, in the form of the microbiome. The biggest problem with antibiotics is that they tend to kill not just the villainous pathogenic bacteria, but the good guys too, which are so important for good health. On the other hand, thanks to antibiotics, people no longer die from small wounds, and doctors can carry out complicated surgeries— so antibiotics have contributed in their own way to longer lifespans. Perhaps even more worrying, however, is the fact that bacteria evolve so quickly that they can develop resistance to the antibiotics faster than we can develop antibiotics to destroy them. Unfortunately, the use of antibiotics is only increasing, not just as prescription medicine, but also to fatten livestock and meat. This means we might soon be dying again from bacterial infections— except this time from bacteria that have, like mutant monsters, become drug-resistant.

Fortunately, the field of immunology is trying to keep up with the zombie bacteria. The French Canadian microbiologist, Félix d'Hérelle, did many interesting things in his life, including bicycling around Europe, investing in a chocolate factory and trying to use maple syrup to make schnapps, but perhaps his most lasting contribution was in the field of microbiology.[4] In 1917, he discovered that certain viruses could infect bacteria and destroy them—he named these 'bacteriophages', literally meaning bacteria eaters. Known as 'phage therapy', this discovery is important in the development of treatments for highly antibiotic-resistant bacteria.

The future of healthcare includes fascinating new ways of harnessing our immune systems to treat serious illness, specifically cancer. Research over the last several years has worked on engineering the body's own immune cells to identify and attack cancer cells and to boost the immune response in the body. Many of these therapies are already in use in treating cancer, while more are currently being researched. Experts believe that these advanced methods could also be applied to other conditions and illnesses.

Auto-Immune Diseases

While our immune system is the best defence we have against the many threats we face every day, it occasionally turns against us. Over-enthusiastic immune cells can start to attack the cells and tissues of our own body, mistakenly identifying them as foreign invaders, resulting in what are known as 'autoimmune diseases'. Around 5 per cent of people, two-thirds of whom are women, suffer from the over fifty different autoimmune diseases that have been identified. Some of the more common ones are type 1 diabetes in which the immune system targets the pancreas-producing cells of the pancreas, rheumatoid arthritis that affects the joints,

Hashimoto's Disease that affects the thyroid and multiple sclerosis that results from damage to the myelin sheaths that protect the cells of the nervous system. As this civil war wages in the body, it is often incredibly difficult to diagnose autoimmune diseases, and, even after diagnosis, treatment is not always wholly effective and can require lifelong medication.

Autoimmune diseases can be terribly debilitating, with symptoms that interfere with normal functioning, and they are found to be far more prevalent in women than men. Unfortunately, we still don't know exactly what causes them. Some theories state that autoimmune diseases could sometimes result from an overreaction of the immune system to an infection or to some form of injury or damage. Still others investigate the role played by genetics, as some of these diseases seem to be heritable to some extent. And finally, recent research has been exploring the links between stress and stress-related disorders on autoimmunity. Even as the field of medicines attempts to unravel the mysteries of autoimmunity, lifestyle modifications can help manage these illnesses.

* * *

'Your lifestyle—how you live, eat, emote, and think—determines your health. To prevent disease, you may have to change how you live.'—Brian Carter

Despite, and perhaps because of, the advances, conveniences and endless streams of information and entertainment in our modern lives, we seem to have created an entirely new class of diseases. The threat to our health doesn't come from an external factor but from how we live our lives. In this chapter we will explore how lifestyle diseases came to be, the toll they exert on the quality of life and what we can do to prevent and even reverse some of them.

WHAT ARE LIFESTYLE DISEASES?

Lifestyle diseases are those caused by the way people live their lives. These ailments are most often the result of the interactions between genetics, physiology, environment and behaviour, and have been found to be caused by one of the following: unhealthy food habits, a lack of physical activity and the use of alcohol, tobacco and drugs. In addition, poor posture, chronic stress and disturbed biological clocks can also cause the symptoms of lifestyle diseases.

The great mismatch between what our bodies evolved to do and what they now do lies at the heart of lifestyle disease.

Some of the most common kinds of lifestyle diseases, also called non-communicable diseases (NCDs), are cardiovascular and chronic respiratory diseases, as well as cancer. Almost all of these, in addition to diabetes, obesity, osteoporosis and polycystic ovarian disease, and to some extent depression, are related to the way we live our lives and the habits we have inculcated. In 2018, the WHO published a fact sheet reporting that NCDs were responsible for 71 per cent of global deaths. A majority of these deaths occurred in middle- and low-income countries and many of them prematurely, between the ages of thirty and sixty-nine. The leading causes of death worldwide are cardiovascular disease, cancers, respiratory diseases and diabetes. In fact, these four types of lifestyle disease accounted for over 80 per cent of premature deaths.

Lifestyle diseases are closely related to metabolic syndrome, a cluster of metabolic factors that includes abdominal obesity (excess fat around the waist), high triglyceride levels, low HDL or good cholesterol, high blood pressure and high fasting blood sugar. If you have three of these five risk factors, you will be diagnosed with metabolic syndrome. Having metabolic syndrome increases your risk for lifestyle diseases like type 2 diabetes, stroke and heart disease. While these metabolic factors are influenced to some extent by genetics and age, they are also affected by a sedentary lifestyle and an unhealthy diet, which are under our control.

The fact that lifestyle diseases are chronic means that they are a huge economic burden on the countries struggling with them. Unlike many other illnesses, they are not time bound and one does not easily recover from them with one-time medication or treatment. In fact, many lifestyle diseases require lifelong medication, cause years of disability and can lead to more health complications. Add to that the fact that some of them seem to be related, such as diabetes, obesity and heart disease, and we truly have a complex group of illnesses on our hands.

Considering the fact that a majority of global deaths are attributed to lifestyle diseases, which have become one of the major threats to health, wellbeing and productivity, we tend to assume that we are helpless in the face of them. We assume that they are an inevitable aspect of modern life and something we just have to learn to live with. However, the thing about our lifestyles is that we get to choose them. In fact, according to the WHO, up to 80 per cent of premature deaths due to heart disease, stroke and diabetes can be prevented.

Apart from genetic predispositions, most of the major factors associated with NCDs are under our control: physical activity, nutrition, sleep and substance abuse. Of course, in some extreme cases, even these might be difficult due to financial or other circumstances, but largely, these are things we can make choices about.

The fact that lifestyle diseases are not inevitable is clear in the stories of how communities that lived in very similar ways to their ancient ancestors had no instances of diabetes, heart disease or cancer, until they were exposed to the 'Western' way of life. In fact, this is why NCDs, until recently, were known as the diseases of civilization or Western diseases.

There are many ways of shifting to a healthier lifestyle, and hopefully, that's what this book will help you figure out. But the first step to protecting ourselves from lifestyle diseases might be simply acknowledging the fact that we don't have to succumb to them as a matter of course.

On the other hand, some lifestyle diseases might not respond to lifestyle changes and that's where things get complex. I have battled high cholesterol since I was in my twenties, and I am beginning to realize that, while this is called a lifestyle disease, it is not something I am able to control with only lifestyle changes. It is likely that, in my case, the condition has genetic underpinnings, while Indians might also be predisposed to high cholesterol and related issues. This has been a source of some frustration for me, because I consider myself largely healthy, I work out regularly and I'm pretty careful with my diet. I have met several doctors and cardiologists and have been prescribed statins to manage my cholesterol. I'm still trying to figure out what lifestyle interventions affect my cholesterol levels and how, but for the time being it seems like a disease I'm going to have to live with—taking medication and monitoring it so that it doesn't get worse. Others might have similar experiences, so it is important not only to try to avoid lifestyle diseases, but to figure out ways of managing and living with them better.

DIABETES

India holds the dubious title of the Diabetes Capital of the world, while the disease has taken on epidemic proportions globally. The common perception of diabetes is that it is a chronic and progressive disease, requiring lifelong medication and often causing other health complications. It is in many ways a debilitating and expensive disease. Fortunately, however, recent research and studies by experts have proved that diabetes is not only preventable, but also reversible. In fact, it is not medication or surgery that will reverse the disease, but changes to lifestyle and diet.

Insulin—a key character in the story of diabetes—is made in the pancreas and released in response to spikes in blood sugar, in order to transport the sugar into the cells of the body to be used as energy. Since the main symptom of diabetes is high levels of sugar in the blood, the assumption is that insulin isn't doing its job right, or that its levels have fallen too low. This is correct in the case of type 1 diabetes, an autoimmune disease in which the insulin-producing cells are destroyed, justifying its treatment with insulin. However, the root cause of type 2 diabetes is too much sugar in the body. In response to this excess glucose, more and more insulin is produced, and, eventually, the cells of the body become resistant to the hormone. As a result, the levels of glucose in the blood continue to build up, leading to the symptoms and risks of type 2 diabetes.

Jason Fung, a nephrologist and the author of the books *The Obesity Code* and *The Diabetes Code*, says that type 2 diabetes is a dietary disease, and the key to preventing it is weight loss. However, type 2 diabetes has almost universally been treated with insulin, which causes weight gain. Clearly, therefore, something isn't quite right with the way we are treating the disease.

Given that diabetes is a *lifestyle* disease, it is also important to treat it with *lifestyle* changes. This starts with a whole foods diet, low in all sugars and refined carbohydrates, but with adequate amounts of protein, fibre and healthy fats. In addition, strong evidence is emerging in favour of fasting as a powerful tool for diabetics. Intermittent and other forms of fasting can help regulate the insulin mechanism. If you suffer from diabetes or borderline diabetes, it is best to consult with your doctor and nutritionist to design meals and eating plans that can help you best manage your condition. Don't forget that exercise can also have a powerful impact on the disease. While you might still be prescribed medication, and should always follow your doctor's advice, don't forget that lifestyle changes could improve and even reverse diabetes.

CARDIOVASCULAR DISEASES

The heart is often likened to the engine that keeps the body going and called the hardest working muscle in the human body. The beating of the heart is synonymous with being alive, as it goes on pumping blood relentlessly throughout our lives, and yet, it is also the organ that can come under tremendous strain due to lifestyle choices. I come from a family where it is routine for people to die in their fifties and sixties from various heart related ailments. Heart disease is growing increasingly common, and it does not discriminate between men and women, rich and poor, old and young. There's no two ways about it—heart disease is killing us. The leading cause of death globally, cardiovascular diseases (CVDs) refer to disorders related to the heart and blood vessels, and include coronary heart disease, cerebrovascular disease and rheumatic heart disease, among many others. Most deaths caused by CVDs occur due to heart attacks and stroke, and a third of these deaths are premature—that is, under the age of seventy.

Considering how prevalent heart disease is, many of us accept it as an inevitable side effect of ageing, genetics or modern life with all its stress. Advances in science and technology mean that people can have machines inserted into them to keep their hearts running, but this also means that heart disease becomes a chronic, lifelong issue. However, just like most other lifestyle diseases, many CVDs are preventable—except those related to inherited disorders or birth defects.

Many long-term health studies have uncovered a profound link between lifestyle, diet in particular, and risk for CVDs. A 2016 review of the famous Nurses Health Study[5] found that a reduced risk for heart disease was related to diets low in refined carbohydrates, sweetened beverages and trans fats, but high in fruits, vegetables, whole grains and unsaturated fats. The lifestyle factors most closely associated with a higher risk for CVDs are smoking, physical inactivity, being overweight and the harmful use of alcohol. A meta-analysis of studies looking into the interactions of lifestyle factors and cardiovascular disease[6] found that adopting several healthy lifestyle behaviours together could reduce risk for CVDs by up to 66 per cent, compared to adopting only one or none.

In many cases, diabetes and obesity are closely linked to heart disease—evidence of an evil nexus between all these lifestyle diseases. On the other hand, a family history of CVDs could also mean that you have an increased risk for these disorders. Regular checkups, in addition to maintaining a healthy body weight, diet, and overall lifestyle, could then be the key to preventing heart disease from taking root.

HYPERTENSION

Hypertension and high blood pressure are terms that have become an integral part of our everyday vocabulary—as in 'don't give me hypertension' or 'this job is going to raise my blood pressure!'—which only serves to point towards the extreme prevalence of this lifestyle disease. Hypertension is the condition in which blood pressure is persistently high. Blood pressure is the force of blood pushing against the walls of the vessels. The higher the pressure, the harder the heart must work to pump blood and the greater the strain on the vessels. Hypertension is diagnosed when, on two different days, systolic pressure is greater than 140 mm/Hg and diastolic pressure is higher than 90 mm/Hg.

Raised blood pressure or hypertension not only increases the burden on the heart as it pumps blood through the body, but also reduces the overall efficiency of this otherwise beautifully synchronized system. Over time, this can damage the tissues lining the arteries, which, in turn, leads to the build-up of plaque and the beginning of atherosclerosis. Atherosclerosis leads to further narrowing of the arteries, which only serves to increase the blood pressure, thus establishing a vicious cycle that often leads to arrhythmia, heart attacks and strokes.

Hypertension is often called the 'silent killer' because those afflicted with it might have no symptoms and no knowledge of the condition, even as damage builds up on the inside. The risk factors for high blood pressure are the same as for most other lifestyle diseases—unhealthy diet, smoking, excessive consumption of alcohol, being overweight or obese and a lack of exercise. There are also factors, such as a family history of hypertension or other existing diseases like diabetes or conditions such as alcohol dependence or obesity. In addition, hypertension can be related to the excessive consumption of caffeine and the use of drugs that could increase blood pressure, including certain non-steroidal anti-inflammatory drugs, glucocorticoids and others. More importantly, however, an increased intake of salt can lead to hypertension, and reduced dietary sodium has been linked to a significantly reduced risk for high blood pressure.

PREVENTING, MANAGING & REVERSING LIFESTYLE DISEASE

While it's great news that most lifestyle diseases can not only be managed but also reversed, the better thing to do is to stay one step ahead of all these chronic ailments. The best news is that this is possible. If you start out with a healthy lifestyle in the first place, it's possible to prevent these diseases from taking root and wreaking havoc with your body and your mind. Much of this book is about doing just that. Developing habits around health, from diet and fitness to meditation and stress management, can truly transform your health journey, protecting you from the epidemic of lifestyle diseases to a great extent. The fact is that there are always some things beyond our control, such as genetics and age, that might make us more vulnerable to certain disorders or diseases. However, there are also many things that are within our control, and we need to make the most of these.

Fortunately for us, the modifiable risk factors for lifestyle disease are all fairly simple to address, and this book will hopefully equip you to do so.

While the prevention, management and reversal of lifestyle diseases might appear simple and straightforward, it can often be far more difficult than it sounds. Adopting a healthier lifestyle might involve rethinking everything about your life so far, changing your relationship with yourself and your body, as well as with food and exercise. This can be a very challenging process and might be best undergone with the guidance of therapists and doctors and the support of family and friends.

HEALTH HACK #22: Take a Walk in Nature

Even if you live in the city, identify one green spot for you to take a nature walk in—a park, a garden, or even a rooftop with a view of the trees. Carve out twenty minutes in your day to take a break and have a 'forest bath'. Leave your devices and gadgets behind and try to truly feel one with nature, experiencing it through all of your senses.

IN SUMMARY

Keep in Mind

1. Immunity is a state of resistance to disease or infection—the immune system is able to differentiate between 'self' and 'non-self' in order to achieve this resistance.
2. The innate immune system is the first line of defence: a generic response activated via the skin, gastric acid, dendritic cells, etc., when a pathogen enters the body.
3. The adaptive immune system response is a learned response: immune cells develop a memory of a pathogen and launch a strategic attack when they encounter it again.
4. Inflammation is the body's way of securing the point of attack with a flood of immune cells, while fever and other symptoms of illness are signs of the immune system at work.
5. The hygiene hypothesis states that the overly sanitized environment of our modern world prevents our children's immune systems from learning through exposure to germs, and this could lead to increased incidence of allergies and autoimmune diseases.
6. Getting a good night's sleep, managing stress through things like meditation, eating nutritious meals, exercising (but not too much) and supplementing when required can help shore up the immune system.
7. Vaccines hack the body's immune response by injecting a small dose of an agent that resembles a pathogen and allows our body to learn how to fight it.
8. Antibiotics inhibit the growth of or destroy harmful bacteria, but in the process, often kill the good microorganisms of the gut.

9. Autoimmune diseases occur when the immune system starts to attack cells and tissues of the body due to one of several conditions, and they disproportionately affect women.

10. Lifestyle diseases are caused by the mismatch between what our bodies evolved to do and what our modern lives require us to do—and many can be traced to unhealthy food habits, lack of physical activity or the use of alcohol, tobacco and drugs.

11. Type 2 diabetes is often thought of as a progressive, chronic, irreversible disorder, but recent studies say that it can be managed with lifestyle changes.

12. Heart disease is the leading cause of death, but we don't have to accept it as our fate or the natural side effects of ageing—instead we can take control of our lifestyles to try and prevent it.

Take Action

1. While you're unwell, practice some light fasting or reduce the portions you eat at every meal. This will free up the energy used for digestion to help you recover.

2. Try and expose yourself to under thirty minutes of sunlight in the morning.

3. Get your vitamin C from natural sources like citrus fruit, papaya, strawberry, cruciferous veggies and leafy greens. If you're really serious about your immunity, speak to your doctor about getting a high-dose injection of vitamin C.

4. Supplement with zinc at the onset of a cold or flu to nip sickness in the bud.

5. If you have been on a course of antibiotics, ask your doctor to prescribe a probiotic to keep your gut happy. Also add pre- and probiotics to your diet during this time.

6. If you've been training hard at the gym and start to feel a bit under the weather, it is possible you haven't taken enough time out for recovery. Take a day off, get a sauna or a massage and give yourself a break before your immune system takes the hit.

7. If you really want to avoid or manage lifestyle diseases, habit change is crucial—especially when it comes to quitting cigarettes, going off alcohol and staying active.

8. Doing regular tests and scans can help you stay one step ahead of lifestyle diseases. If you know if you have a genetic predisposition for these diseases, it is even more important to keep an eye on the risk factors.

9. Cut down on your sugar consumption to prevent or reverse metabolic syndrome, which is highly correlated with most lifestyle diseases.

9

MANAGING
MENTAL HEALTH

In the depths of winter, I finally learned that within me is an invincible summer.— Albert Camus

Every family is strange in its own way, and growing up, my family was no different. Some of my relatives had what I then thought was the rather odd habit of getting 'possessed' by what were assumed to be deities. This tended to happen during large gatherings or particularly stressful situations, I noticed. Their demeanour and facial expressions would suddenly change; eyes rolling in their sockets, voices turning hoarse as their bodies began to shake uncontrollably and vigorously. This was a terrifying sight for us children, and for the grown-ups, this caused a great deal of commotion. I observed how the adults would rush to the conclusion that the person in question had been possessed by some divine power. To appease the god or goddess who had suddenly descended to earth and to fulfil their demands, certain rituals would need to be conducted. Thus, various ceremonies would take place and the divine powers would be placated, but my young brain was left confused and scared—not knowing what had just happened or how to process it.

Now that I have a better understanding of mental health, I have begun to wonder if these situations weren't, in fact, an expression of an underlying illness. Perhaps the possession was a form of paranoia induced by extreme stress, or an outlet for a person whose mental health was suffering. I've come to realize that due to the taboo and shame associated with mental health, many illnesses have not only gone undiagnosed and untreated, but have also been explained away with various reasons, including divine powers.

While greater awareness now exists and better solutions in terms of medication and therapy are available, we are also witnessing an alarming rise in mental health issues. From anxiety and depression to sleep disorders, mental illness seems to be pervasive, and still only a small number of people seek help. The field is in urgent need of attention, as mental health might have an even greater impact on quality of life than most physical ailments. We simply cannot afford to ignore this growing pandemic, and in this chapter, we try to shine some light on mental health and its management.

MENTAL HEALTH AND STIGMA

While conversations on health are coming into the mainstream, in the office and online, through books and documentaries, one aspect remains in the shadows. If you get injured or fall ill, sympathy and offers of support pour in from all quarters. You can get paid time off from work and are likely to receive recommendations for a host of relevant health experts. The same understanding doesn't extend to mental health, however, and millions pay the price as a result. It isn't uncommon for someone feeling low or depressed to be offered the 'friendly' advice to 'cheer up' or 'look on the bright side'—in effect, brushing off what could be a deeper issue. We would never tell someone with a broken leg to 'be a good sport' or to 'just walk'. Not only do people living with mental illness struggle with the disease itself, but they also face derision and mistreatment, often being ostracized by society. The stigma associated with mental health is a tragedy, but fortunately, things are gradually changing.

With advances in research, more books being published on the subject and several public figures opening up about their own struggles, awareness is increasing and there is more open discourse on the topic. In addition, there has been a proliferation of options to support better mental health, from meditation, yoga and therapy to medication. We still have a long way to go, especially in India, but hopefully, we're on the right track.

Mental health is complex; made more complex by how extraordinarily unique each of us is, not only in the way our brains are wired, but also in how we feel, think, process and respond to different situations. It also isn't easy to 'measure' mental health because so much of it is subjective and dependent on thoughts and emotions. Despite extensively researched diagnostic manuals, it also isn't easy to diagnose mental health disorders. And while I can give you tips for fitness and food, because movement is largely good for you and refined sugar is largely bad for you, when it comes to mental health, there are no generic hacks or simple solutions. What works for someone else might not work for you, and that's just fine.

Personally, when the stress or anxiety of work starts getting to me, I take a break and hit the gym to help reset my mind and body. For someone else, just the thought of getting out of bed and going to the gym can be too overwhelming to even contemplate. While an overall healthy lifestyle can boost mental wellness, you might be the fittest, healthiest eater with great habits, and you might still struggle with depression or anxiety. There are no easy answers for mental health, but fortunately, with advances in science and medicine, we now have many more options than we did before. For some, dietary changes could have a positive impact on mental health, while for others, therapy and medication or breathwork and meditation could make all the difference.

The most important thing when it comes to mental health, though, could be the ability to have open conversations without fear of shame or judgement. To be able to discuss our mental health and our struggles with family, friends, doctors and others can be the first step towards greater awareness and acceptance, and finally, healing. But even this is easier said than done, as most forms of depression make you want to hide or just be alone. It is difficult to muster the courage and energy to even begin the conversation with close family members. Having caring and patient people around, who can infer what's going on and encourage the person in question to gradually open up and seek help, can go a long way in treating the condition.

WHAT IS MENTAL HEALTH?

Mental health is often defined as emotional, psychological and social wellbeing. The first Director-General of the WHO, Dr Brock Chisholm was a psychiatrist who said, '. . . without mental health there can be no true physical health'.[1] And I would like to add that the reverse is absolutely true as well, further reinforcing the mind–body connection that we have only just begun to understand. This points to the importance of mental health in ensuring a good quality of life—being able to sustain relationships, actively engage in work and other pursuits, and develop resilience to life's ups and downs.

Over the course of their lives, many people might experience mental health problems of various kinds and to different degrees. These problems can interfere with one's mood, behaviour, and thought processes, having a negative impact on day-to-day activities. Most mental illnesses aren't caused by a single factor or life event and are often a result of a combination of things, including genetics or a family history of mental health problems, lifestyle or life experiences and brain chemistry or circuitry. Having a high stress job or going through a personal trauma of some sort can make you more vulnerable to certain mental illnesses. Recent research into the gut as the body's second brain has also raised questions about the role of gastrointestinal problems in the diagnosis and treatment of mental illnesses.

In his book *The End of Mental Illness*, Daniel Amen argues for the reframing of mental health as 'brain health' to shift the conversation from the 'moral' to the 'medical'. He finds the current diagnostic paradigm inadequate and suggests a comprehensive and holistic approach to the field that considers what he calls the 'four circles'—biological, psychological, social and spiritual. In his work with patients, Amen has found certain risk factors in common, which he has nicknamed BRIGHT MINDS: Blood Flow, Retirement/ Ageing, Inflammation, Genetics, Head Trauma, Toxins, Mindstorms, Immunity/ Infections, Neurohormone Issues, Diabesity, and Sleep. For example, exposure to environmental toxins—from cleaning and beauty products, paint or other chemicals—could cause significant damage to the brain and lead to one of several mental health disorders. In addition, even a history of infectious diseases could make us more vulnerable to certain mental health disorders. Therefore, he firmly believes that, while genetics and family history do play a role in the expression of disorders, caring for one's overall brain and body, taking steps to improve one's environment and lifestyle, and regularly testing for various health markers, can be a big step towards more effectively treating problems of mental health.

Very often we think of anything related to mental health as extreme and abnormal, but increasingly, the conversation is shifting to the idea of a spectrum that we all inhabit. Every one of us will experience feelings of anxiety, sadness, depression, or outbursts of anger and irritation at some points in our lives. After all, to be human is to experience emotions. However, when these emotions begin to interfere with our functioning in our daily lives, or when we are struggling to cope with them, we might be diagnosed with a mental health disorder that requires intervention in some form. When we can see that we all share several of these symptoms, and that 'normal' is a relative term, perhaps we will be able to experience a world that is truly more inclusive, accepting and kind.

The Diagnostic and Statistical Manual (DSM), developed by the American Psychiatric Association and now in its fifth edition, attempts to categorize all disorders of mental health. While standardization can be useful, and the DSM has helped to guide research and development of therapy options, there are also several drawbacks to this approach. One major disadvantage is that human behaviour is a complex thing, occurring on a continuum of sorts, so definitions of mental health tend towards oversimplification. In addition, since there is often a vast overlap of symptoms between disorders, misdiagnoses become common. The labels defined in the DSM are not only attached to stigma, but also lead to overdiagnosis—when someone's behaviour doesn't fit in with what is considered 'normal' or 'ideal'.

On the other hand, for people who have been struggling for years without knowing how to navigate their circumstances, a diagnosis might offer clarity on how to move forward with treatment and healing. Mental health professionals continue to use the DSM as a useful tool in their work. In the words of some experts, the DSM is 'a dictionary, not a bible' to refer to, while allowing conversations with patients to lead the way.

Unfortunately, when it comes to mental health 'disorders' or 'illnesses', our very first response is to approach them as some sort of deficiency. As a result, we assume there is something fundamentally wrong with us if we struggle with our mental health, and are plagued by feelings of shame and guilt for who we are. However, people are increasingly trying to change the lens through which we view problems related to mental health. In his fascinating book *The Depths: The Evolutionary Origins of the Depression Epidemic,* Jonathan Rottenberg rejects this tendency to blame depression on a faulty way of thinking or a faulty brain, offering instead a way of looking at it through affective science or the science of mood. He claims that mood systems—which relate to depression, anxiety, and other so-called disorders—have their roots in evolutionary adaptations and, like every other adaptation, have their pros and cons. For example, low moods could help de-escalate conflict which might have increased survival, or prevent one from persisting in a situation that might have been dangerous or led to a waste of energy.

It's okay to not be okay

While mental health has been a subject of taboo for most of us, those in the media spotlight face even more pressure to appear okay even when they are not. This is why 2021 was a landmark year for mental health in the field of sports. Tennis player Naomi Osaka decided to skip a press conference at the French Open to take care of her mental health, a move that led to much scrutiny and criticism. However, many came out in support of her, inspiring a conversation about the hidden mental health struggles that athletes face. Weeks later, gymnastic superstar Simone Biles pulled out of the women's team final at the Tokyo Olympics so she could focus on her mental health. Soon after, cricketer Ben Stokes announced that he would be taking a break to prioritize his mental health. For famous athletes, the pressure to win and achieve traditional ideas of success is enormous. As a result, many of them battle with anxiety, stress and other disorders. There is also very little compassion extended to them in this regard, as they are expected to fulfil their roles as public figures—playing to the media and audiences, acting as if they are okay when they are not. Hopefully, Osaka, Biles and Stokes are changing the dialogue around mental health in the public sphere.

Just as we can boost our physical resilience to prevent ourselves from falling sick too often, it might also be possible to shore up our mental health. And the surprising thing—or perhaps not so surprising, given what we know about the mind–body connection—is that this first line of defence looks similar in both cases. Therefore, having a fairly good routine that includes a nutritious diet, some exercise, good sleep, and social support can help us stay not just physically but also mentally well. The fact is that when we struggle with low moods, anxiety or even stress, these fundamentals tend to be the first victims–and that's okay, even normal. But if homemade food or a daily walk with a friend are already integral parts of your day—part of a routine that feels comfortable and familiar—then you are more likely to stick to these healthier habits, even when the going gets tough. And these can make you more resilient to the challenges you face.

Whatever the theories put forward for problems of mental health, most agree on one thing: that the most fundamental flaw in our thinking has been to see them as deficiencies, and this is what has led to years of stigma, judgement, and feelings of inadequacy. Reframing the issue, therefore, might be the most pivotal change we can make in our approach to this field. Equipped with a sound understanding of what mental health is, how it works, and how it can influence our lives, mindsets, and personalities, can help us leverage the advances in medicine and technology that can help us find true health, not just of body, but of mind as well.

FEELING & THINKING

As much as we exist in the real, tangible world, so much of what we do is driven by our interior world—thoughts, emotions, memories of the past, visions of the future. Much like the one around us, our interior landscape is constantly shifting and evolving. And while these fluctuations in mood are normal and in fact essential to the human experience, we actually might have more control over our emotions than we previously thought. This doesn't mean that we can't still be knocked down by feelings of inadequacy or worries about what may or may not happen tomorrow. But the knowledge that we aren't completely at the mercy of our emotions can be empowering, considering how much turmoil they often cause.

One of the simplest yet profound ideas that therapy often teaches is that you are not defined by your emotions or thoughts—these are things you experience, not who you are. Our feelings and moods are not just a reflection of what's going on in our heads, but the result of a complex and constant feedback loop between our bodies, environments, and lifestyles and how our brains interpret all this information. Many therapists include questions about where you feel certain emotions or moods in your body—for example, does anxiety manifest as a knotted neck, or depression as a pit in your stomach? They might also ask questions about your past, your relationships, and your daily habits, because all this feeds into your mood and state of mental health.

When we experience a negative emotion, our first reaction is usually to suppress it. We often escape through activities that give us instant gratification because they numb uncomfortable feelings. The distraction is momentary, however, and not only do we indulge in unhealthy habits in the process, but we also get caught in a vicious cycle because we can't really outrun our feelings.

Our thoughts can sometimes feel overwhelming—bigger than us even. When we're feeling low or anxious, we are consumed by negative thoughts. Fortunately for us, the same brains that make it possible for us to get stuck in these loops also have an incredible skill known as metacognition—literally, thinking about one's thinking. Therapy harnesses this ability, building self-awareness so that we are better able to separate ourselves from our thoughts, emotions, and moods. This distance gives us a moment of pause and allows us to gain perspective, recognizing that thoughts and emotions, especially negative ones, are not the result of a fault in the brain, but are the brain's way of processing information.

The mind is a wonderfully complex thing, and I often find it fascinating to observe the ways in which it works—even when it is seemingly working against us. One way in which this happens, especially when we're feeling depressed or anxious, is through what are known as cognitive biases, shortcuts that the brain relies on to save time and effort. We might rely on a mental filter or confirmation bias, which scans the evidence and spotlights only that which confirms what we already believe. For example, if you are convinced that you're terrible at your job, you might ignore the high rating you received in your last review and instead pick out only those moments that you perceive as failures. Another common bias is overgeneralization, when we let one low point define the entire day, convinced nothing can make it better. We also tend to personalize and catastrophize more than usual if we're feeling anxious or low.

Growing aware of the thoughts and emotions that we get caught up in or recognizing the biases we have fallen for can help us take our mental wellbeing into our own hands. Therapy is one route, and another potent tool is mindfulness. Mindfulness cultivates a deep sense of self-awareness without judgement or action. A mindful attitude allows you to observe emotions without immediately responding to or acting on them. With a curious mind, you can label the emotion washing over you, looking at the bigger picture instead of getting tangled up in it. Creating this gap or this pause can give your brain the time it needs to choose a response more thoughtfully than if you get swept up in big feelings. Incorporating a mindful practice in our daily life has many benefits, but one of its greatest impacts is on the way we handle our thoughts and emotions for better mental health.

I have found that being conscious of where I spend my attention helps me keep my eye on the bigger picture, making it easier to handle difficult thoughts and emotions. Mindfulness also helps us consciously redirect our attention, something that is crucial in a world where it is easy to lose track and get disconnected. Reconnecting with our core values can lend our days purpose and motivation.

Despite learning about how your brain works and developing self-awareness, it is still difficult to slow down and be mindful when you're not feeling your best. And that's OK. What could help is journaling everything you can remember about that moment of struggle after it has passed—the thoughts that went through your mind, the feelings that washed over you, the way your body felt, and the thing that finally helped you calm down. In her fantastic book *Why Has Nobody Ever Told Me This Before*, clinical psychologist Dr Julie Smith suggests trying to separate thoughts, emotions, physical sensations and behaviours from each other, to observe how each affects the other. After observing these four aspects closely, ask yourself what thoughts and emotions you would like to have instead, what sensations you would welcome in your body, and how you would ideally like to behave.

There are so many tools from the various kinds of therapy that we can pick from to build an arsenal for better emotional resilience and mental health. And yet, there might continue to be occasions when your mood or your anxiety, your thoughts, and feelings, strike you down. The process has ups and downs, and more than anything, it is important to be kind, honest and compassionate with yourself, as you seek help and navigate your own, unique mental health journey.

DEALING WITH STRESS

Before we go any further, it's important to acknowledge the role that stress plays in health, particularly of the mind. Stress has been defined as the physiological response to a stressor, something in the environment that disrupts the body's homeostasis. The stress response, therefore, attempts to re-establish balance in the body. If the body and mind have enough resources on hand, they can counter demands placed on them by the stressor. It is when resources are insufficient that its negative effects on health take root.

For most living creatures, stress is a response to a short-lived, immediate, acute threat—such as being chased by a predator. In this case, stress not only alerts us to a threat in our environment, but also prepares the body through the release of hormones and activation of the nervous system, among other physiological changes, to face the stressor. However, thanks to the extraordinarily different circumstances in which we live compared to the environment we evolved in as homo sapiens, there is a massive disconnect between the nature of the stressor, and the body's response to it. In other words, we misconstrue an all caps email reply as a threat which triggers an increase in heart rate, blood pressure and cortisol, just like we would when we face a predator in the wild!

Much of the stress we experience in our lives today emerges from disruptions to our psychological and social wellbeing. In addition, the complexity of our brains and our ability to think about the future means that sometimes even the anticipation of an event, or the possibility of a disruption, can cause stress. Therefore, neither is the stress acute, nor does it pose an immediate threat to our physical wellbeing. Yet the body is constantly preparing itself to go into full fight mode. Thus, our bodies and minds are constantly on alert, ready for action, even when there isn't a tangible, real-life stressor—only one that is in our heads or in the distant future.

In addition, our brains and bodies expect to receive a reward after a period of stress—the equivalent of a feast after a successful hunting expedition. However, instead of some much needed R&R and downtime, our modern lives often keep us in a constant state of stress. And this is what makes stress dangerous, taking a toll on our physical and mental health, making us more vulnerable to illnesses, affecting our moods, our ability to make decisions and control our impulses.

A Languishing State of Affairs

The COVID-19 pandemic affected people's mental health in many ways, but one that psychologist and author Adam Grant identified as the 'dominant emotion' of 2021, is languishing. Somewhere in between thriving or flourishing and being depressed, is this feeling of emptiness—marked by a lack of motivation and an inability to focus on work. Descending into a state of indifference with nothing to look forward to, those who are languishing might not even notice that something isn't right and therefore do not seek help. As a result, languishing, which might not be categorized as a mental illness, can lead to more serious disorders. According to Grant, identifying and naming this state is a first step towards improving it. Moments of flow, in which we are fully immersed in an activity that challenges and excites us, periods of time without interruptions, and focusing on small wins might be ways of combating that feeling of languishing.

Dealing with stress can be particularly tricky because of how dramatically stressors vary in type and intensity, and how differently each of us responds to them. What is stressful to me, for example, might not cause you stress. Some of the most common stressors in our modern lives, however, are meeting deadlines, juggling professional demands with personal ones, facing financial pressures, and experiencing caregiver stress. Stressors are commonly categorized as financial (which includes being in debt), physical (including illness, overtraining, lack of sleep), emotional (such as shame or guilt), environmental (which could be noise and other pollution) as well as cultural (such as homesickness).

Considering how common stress has become, you might when to take action or seek help to counter its negative effects. While it might be a good idea to address sources of stress as soon as you notice them, stress can affect us at different levels, and it is important to pay attention and to listen to your body and your mind. When life is not challenging enough—lacking in healthy stress—you might feel slightly lethargic, bored or unfocused. With just the right amount of stress or challenge, however, you will feel energized; as though you are constantly moving towards your goals, constantly learning and growing. Known as eustress, this keeps us going and motivates us to try our best to tackle problems or challenges. With high levels of stress, however, feelings of anxiety and helplessness might be experienced. Chronic stress can affect your day-to-day functioning, leaving you feeling fatigued and overburdened. Often, chronic stress is accompanied by digestive and hormonal issues, an inability to sleep or concentrate at work, a tendency to turn to alcohol, smoking or binge eating as coping mechanisms, and avoidance behaviours towards even manageable stress, leaving your body and mind out of balance.

Just as controlled stress such as exercise is good for the body, studies have found that not all stress is bad for the mind. Stress is that wild energy that can destroy you if left uncontrolled but if tamed and used judiciously, can be a source of continued growth in your life. There are stressors in our lives that are unavoidable, such as unexpected financial or family struggles, so rather than avoiding all stress which is unrealistic, it is more important to learn how to manage our response to it. In fact, if you think about it, we are most stressed out by the things that are most important to us—relationships, life goals, financial stability or big events. Learning how to better approach stress can help us leverage its benefits without allowing it to become chronic. The positive effects of stress are often related to an individual's perception or attitude towards stress.

When we talk about the effects of stress, most of us talk about the release of the hormone cortisol and its negative effects, or of adrenaline and its role in mobilizing the body's resources. However, there is another stress hormone, also released by the adrenal glands, called dehydroepiandrosterone (DHEA). While cortisol helps mobilize energy to handle stressful situations and to suppress biological functions such as digestion and growth, DHEA is a neurosteroid that is a precursor for other hormones, also acting as a counter to some of the effects of cortisol. While cortisol is linked to poor immune function and depression, among other things, DHEA released in the right amount has been found to boost brain growth, enhance immunity, and reduce the risk of anxiety, depression and heart disease. While both hormones have important roles in the body, there is a delicate balance or ratio between the two that determines the long-term effects of stress. This is known as the growth index of the stress response, and the more DHEA in relation to cortisol, the more people flourish when under stress. A better growth index—that is higher levels of DHEA—predicts better resilience, persistence and recovery even from extreme stress.

Knowing that our response to stress might be more in our control than we think can be empowering. And sometimes, the simplest things can make all the difference. Studies have recently proven that even a small amount of time spent in nature can have a positive impact on our health and wellbeing. And perhaps this is why doctors these days are prescribing nature for a host of ailments, most related to stress.

The Japanese have coined the term Shinrin-yoku, which translates to Forest Bathing or 'taking in the forest atmosphere'. To take a forest bath all you need to do is identify a spot surrounded by trees and greenery. All devices and technology must be left behind so that you can enjoy the experience without any distraction. In Shinrin-yoku, one uses every sense: seeing the different shades of green, listening to birdsong or the sounds of the wind rustling through the trees, smelling the fragrance of fresh earth, tasting the fresh air as you inhale, and touching the bark of a tree, the soft blades of grass, or dipping your toes in a river.

A 2015 study conducted in Japan on middle-aged males found that Forest Bathing reduced pulse rate, as well as reduced feelings of fatigue, depression and anxiety. A similar study looked at the effects of a two-day Shinrin-yoku programme on middle-aged females in Taiwan, specifically at its role in stress recovery. The researchers found that not only did the subjects report decreases in negative mood states such as fatigue, depression and confusion, but also significant reductions in systolic blood pressure.

The other way of combating stress might be even simpler: spending time with friends and family. Having social support or a strong community around you has been found not only to help alleviate stress but is also associated with better health and lower rates of mortality. We live in a time of rising loneliness. Our devices are always stealing our attention from real life interactions, we often live far from home and our families, and making friends only grows harder with age. Now, more than ever, we need to invest in strong and healthy relationships.

The effects of social support appear to be linked to sympathetic nervous system activity—which is at the heart of the stress response. In laboratory stress tests, participants who have the support of one other person experience significantly lower increases in heart rate, blood pressure and cortisol levels than those working in isolation. Other studies have discovered that oxytocin—the hormone involved in social bonding—might play a role in inhibiting the stress response. People with higher levels of oxytocin and with access to social support report less anxiety and have lower levels of cortisol. Therefore, when we can reach out to our community, oxytocin levels are boosted and, in response, sympathetic activation is subdued.

Breathing techniques can have a profound impact on the physiological stress response. Slowing the breath while extending exhalations has an actual effect on the nervous system, switching from fight or flight to a calmer state. A therapist might also offer different tools to help you alter your relationship with stress, including ways of reframing stressful situations or rethinking your approach to failure. A growth mindset, or one in which you are open to making mistakes and learning from them, fosters a positive relationship with stress, and this is something a therapist could help you cultivate.

Stress management is a fundamental aspect of any health journey—whether this means trying to avoid sources of stress, attempting to adopt a more positive approach to it, or finding ways to de-stress.

ANXIETY & DEPRESSION

My life has been full of terrible misfortunes, most of which never happened.— Michel de Montaigne

While mental health lies on a spectrum and psychiatry has identified several disorders, two of the most common illnesses we struggle with in the modern world are anxiety and depression. Anxiety is a normal reaction to a situation that appears to threaten us. However, when feelings of anxiety or nervousness are disproportionate to the circumstances, persistent and excessive, and when they lead to behaviours that interfere with normal day-to-day function, an anxiety disorder might be diagnosed. There are several types of anxiety disorders, including generalized anxiety disorder, panic disorder which is characterized by panic attacks, phobias, separation anxiety disorder, and social anxiety disorder.

People living with anxiety disorders might go out of their way to avoid situations that trigger them, and this often leads to serious problems with their everyday lives, at school or at work. They might feel constantly restless, tense or nervous, find it hard to concentrate, and might also have a sense of impending doom. These could be accompanied by physical symptoms such as breathlessness or hyperventilation, sweating, trembling, insomnia, and gastrointestinal problems.

The parts of the brain involved in some mental health problems, such as anxiety and depression, are the executive centre, which is the prefrontal cortex or the thinking brain, and the more ancient limbic system, consisting of the hypothalamus, amygdala, hippocampus and cingulate cortex, known as the feeling brain. Anxiety is believed to be caused by a combination of factors, influenced by genetics, environment, lifestyle and brain chemistry. A person might have a history of anxiety disorders in the family, and a traumatic experience might trigger the excessive anxious response. Some studies show that the neurotransmitter GABA plays a role in regulating the anxiety response. People with anxiety disorders also seem to hyperactivate the amygdala—the part of the brain involved in fear responses and emotional regulation—while the regulatory control of the prefrontal cortex is hypoactive.

Interestingly, the brains of anxious and non-anxious people while worrying look pretty much identical—the problem seems to be that people with anxiety are unable to, in a sense, turn off the worry button. The same part of the human brain that allows us to plan for the future, solve complicated problems and achieve other kinds of complex thought, also makes us vulnerable to worrying.

Unfortunately, while worrying about something is occasionally useful—like when it keeps you studying for a big exam or working to meet a deadline—it often wreaks havoc with our days . . . and nights too. Worry can prevent you from applying your mind at work or from staying present and enjoying a moment with your family. It can leave you feeling drained, prevent you from getting a good night's sleep and even lead to depression.

Depression (also called major depressive disorder) can have a deep negative impact on your life and function. It affects how you feel, think and behave, and makes ordinary functioning at home and at work extremely challenging. And yet, we still don't know with complete certainty what exactly causes depression. The brain of a depressed person doesn't have any significant difference from that of a person without depression. All of us tend to occasionally feel sad, but we also have a tendency for positivity that balances this out. However, for some people, the sadness seems to lead them down a spiral of negativity and a persistently depressed mood, which eventually interferes with their ability to function in the world.

People living with depression are sometimes told by (well-meaning) family and friends to 'snap out of it' or to 'pull up their socks', but the fact is that people living with it are doing the best they can and are struggling. From the disease point of view of mental health, they are suffering from an illness that requires intervention and treatment that is often long term. And if we're looking at it in terms of just having a brain that is wired differently, then too depression requires a form of rewiring the brain to address the symptoms—especially when they become debilitating.

Interestingly, depression is also considered a lifestyle disease. This is because a vicious cycle seems to exist between depression and lifestyle habits—depression exacerbates unhealthy behaviours, while those with unhealthy lifestyles are more at risk for developing depression.

Mental Health Beyond Humans

As much as we humans like to think of ourselves as special, with unique emotional and psychological experiences, studies are finding that animals might suffer from mental illness too. For example, research shows that rats and monkeys raised in isolation show symptoms of depression, including a loss of interest in pleasurable activities and an inability to focus on activities. Some believe that animals experience a similar variety, richness and depth of emotion as humans do—from grief and courage to revenge. As a result, they might also suffer disorders that might resemble homesickness, anxiety and obsessive compulsiveness. This isn't so surprising when one thinks back to the fact that almost all emotions played an evolutionary role. Acknowledging this fact can help us understand the animals in our lives better—from pets to those we encounter in the wild—but can also offer us insight into our own experiences with mental health.

We all feel sad and experience grief at various points in our lives—when we lose a family member or friend, lose a job, or experience the end of a relationship. However, although depression is characterized by feeling sad and depressed, it is clinically defined as having one of the following symptoms consistently for a period of at least two weeks: a loss of interest in activities previously enjoyed, changes in appetite or weight and eating patterns, insomnia or a desire to sleep excessively, fatigue or a lack of energy, obvious restlessness or a slowing down of behaviour, feelings of guilt or worthlessness, an inability to concentrate or make decisions and thoughts of death or suicide.

Many mothers suffer from postpartum depression shortly after giving birth—a mental health issue that is severely underdiagnosed. Characterized by feelings of emptiness, sadness and a lack of connection with the baby, many women endure postpartum depression alone and in silence because of the social stigma attached to it, even now. New mums are expected to be ecstatic about their babies, but the fact is that several have a traumatic time—and yet, due to a lack of awareness and the taboo, they cannot seek the help they need. Postpartum depression is believed to be caused by extreme hormonal changes after giving birth, fatigue or pain, a lack of sleep, as well as feelings of self-doubt and loss after giving birth. Without the proper diagnosis and treatment, postpartum depression can lead to distressed families, and even suicide. Unfortunately, even in the field of mental health, research into women's health seems to take a backseat. Open conversations with your doctor, combined with a robust social support system can help with early diagnosis of postpartum depression, while treatment could include therapy and medication. While, increasingly, there is a growing dialogue around postpartum depression, there are other mental health issues that women struggle with that are rarely given attention, including the changes women undergo post menopause. The changes women experience in their bodies and hormonal levels often have profound effects on their state of mental health. A lack of awareness means that these problems often go undiagnosed or untreated.

Like most other mental illnesses, depression is a result of a combination of factors. One of the most commonly accepted theories is that it is related to an imbalance of neurotransmitters including dopamine, serotonin and norepinephrine. Serotonin is involved in mood regulation and willpower, dopamine is the neurotransmitter responsible for motivation and drive, while norepinephrine plays a role in the stress response and staying alert or aroused. In addition, several others are part of the intricate symphony of neurotransmitters that keep our moods stable. These include oxytocin, which promotes trust and love; GABA, which reduces anxiety and increases relaxation; melatonin, that plays an important role in sleep quality; endorphins, which are related to pain relief and that familiar feeling of elation after a run; and endocannabinoids, that are involved in appetite and overall feelings of wellbeing. Changes in activity and levels of these chemicals are associated with depression—explaining the mood swings, feelings of sadness, and lack of interest in previously pleasurable activities.

The parts of the brain that play a role in depression are similar to those in anxiety. The prefrontal cortex, one of the most recently developed regions, gives us a huge evolutionary advantage, but is also one of the reasons we feel guilt, shame, worry and indecisiveness. The hypothalamus, which raises stress hormones, is overactive in people with depression, leading to a constant state of tension. The amygdala too, closely related to the fight-or-flight response and anxiety, is always on high alert.

The hippocampus, which plays a crucial role in memory and is context dependent, might lead to a focus on negative rather than happy memories. In depressed people, the wiring of the cingulate cortex, where serotonin is concentrated, might lead to a difficulty in paying attention.

In addition to chemical imbalances and brain circuitry, depression is also closely linked to genetics—studies have found that the twin of a person living with this mental illness has a 70 per cent chance of having it too. There are also certain dimensions of personality (a lack of self-esteem, an inability to be optimistic) and environment (neglect or abuse in early childhood) that could make a person more vulnerable to depression. Most significantly, perhaps, recent research has brought the spotlight on the intimate connection between our gut and our moods, linking depression to gut health. The fact that antidepressants have been successfully used in the treatment of irritable bowel syndrome or IBS is a powerful illustration of this. The brain–gut–microbiota axis, as it is called, is the subject of some fascinating new studies that might offer us an entirely new perspective on mental health and its management. It might be important to pay attention to our digestive health, especially when we observe changes in our state of mind.

DEALING WITH TRAUMA

The English philosopher Thomas Hobbes observed in the sixteenth century that human life is 'solitary, poor, nasty, brutish and short'.[2] While this may sound like a rather harsh characterization of our life, the truth is that life is certainly not a bed of roses for anyone. Most people suffer from one traumatic event or another during their lives. It can be the sudden death of a loved one, a major accident, a significant financial setback, debilitating diseases, dysfunctional relationships or a history of abuse. We may think of these traumatic events as just part and parcel of life and believe that we know how to handle them, but if you think about it, no one ever really teaches us the best coping strategies to deal with traumatic events. If untreated or not managed well, these traumatic events can result in deep psychological scars with biological footprints in the psyche and body and can continue to trigger a variety of mental health issues throughout one's life.

Psychologist and author Bessel van der Kolk has written an outstanding book on trauma and healing, called *The Body Keeps the Score*. Kolk talks about how traumatic experiences shape us and continue to plague us often even decades after the event. He cites the example of a pregnant mother driving with her five-year-old daughter. The mother gets distracted and runs a redlight which results in another car smashing into hers, instantly killing her daughter. On her way to the ER, she has a miscarriage as well. She enters a near catatonic state after this tragic event and loses all ability to function in social settings. Even the sight or sound of little children would trigger a deep panic and until her treatment with Kolk, she had to live a highly suffocated life.[3]

Many people suffer very difficult situations as children—whether the loss of a parent, abuse, or being brutally bullied at school. These experiences trigger profound changes in the body to cope with the situation. In order to cope, people usually exist in a state of denial, parking the memory in some distant corner of the mind and adopting an exterior façade to project a different image altogether. As a result, people often inadvertently adopt a dissociated personality that is not an integral whole. While these might help as temporary protection mechanisms, they do cause deep long term personality challenges which come in the way of pursuing a happy and fulfilling life.

During every traumatic event, our senses heighten which leads to the memory of the event getting deeply etched into our brains. For example, most people in the US remember exactly what they were doing on the day of 11 September 2001, but no one remembers what they did on 10 September 2001. It is said that 'emotional memories are forever'. And sometimes this quirk of the brain, that no doubt had evolutionary advantages, can lead to some intense but fragmented trauma memories, which, if not resolved, can continue to disrupt the rhythm of life for the affected person.

Therapists like Kolk work with their patients to gradually go back to the past, recall what really happened, what it made the person feel and how they would have liked the situation to be very different in an alternate world. Sometimes talking about the past and revisiting a traumatic memory is too difficult and in these cases, a therapist might employ various calming techniques ranging from body work, neuro-feedback and dance therapy to eye-movement-desensitization and reprioritization (EMDR) techniques to make the patient get comfortable enough to reprocess and come to terms with the source of trauma.

We have come a long way, however, and now recognize many trauma disorders such as PTSD (post traumatic stress disorder) which can be caused by exposure to violence, a history of abuse, and even difficult relationships such as being the partner of a narcissist. PTSD is also common among war veterans who are exposed to death and brutality on the field. As recently as the Vietnam War, the troubled mental state of returning American soldiers was attributed to a weak personality and not given much attention. Things have changed considerably now and people suffering from PTSD can get proper treatment and therapies to cope with the intense stress and subsequent personality changes that are triggered by the experience.

Toxic Positivity & the Dangers of Wellness Culture

Much of the social media conversation these days centres on the idea of 'positive vibes only'. We are bombarded by messaging that tells us to just stay positive and everything will be fine. Positive affirmations, we're told, will magically manifest the life of our dreams. Everywhere we look, we see images and messages of people who are always happy, and we are made to believe that eternal happiness is achievable and, in fact, desirable. At first glance, there's nothing wrong with all this positivity and joy doing the rounds. But dig a little deeper, and you see why it could be problematic, especially at a time when so many of us are struggling with our mental health.

The focus on positivity can make those who are experiencing low moods feel inadequate—as though their inability to feel happy is the result of a faulty brain. When you're told to 'just be positive' and then you find yourself unable to feel positive, you might feel worse. Your negativity becomes a reason for you to criticize yourself and feel as though you have failed to achieve what seems to be well within everyone's reach. Propagating an image of eternal happiness is also simply misleading—nobody can be happy all the time. But Instagram tells you otherwise so that, when you don't feel happy, you become convinced there's something wrong with you. If you can't be happy like everyone else seems to be, you probably have a mental health problem, right? But that's far from the truth. We know that our moods, thoughts and emotions are constantly changing, going up and down depending on myriad factors.

In a 2021 article, social psychologist Dr Tom Curran, who specializes in perfectionism, warns against the unrealistic standards we set ourselves and the punishing methods of achieving them that we submit to. The reason we become perfectionists is because we believe that we are fundamentally lacking in some way, but unfortunately, the pursuit of perfection often only leads to stress, anxiety and obsessive behaviours. The wellness culture taps into this vicious cycle, often selling you expensive and stylish products as well, from detox cleanses to green juices to unique meditation or exercise classes. You spend thousands of your hard-earned rupees on all of this, and instead of feeling well, you end up feeling worse—a failure who is unable to be happy all the time, despite using all these so-called miracle pills and rituals.

Another aspect of this culture is the idea of positive affirmations— that if you keep repeating something to yourself, you will become it. Unfortunately, studies have found that for people with low self-esteem, repeating statements they think are untrue makes them feel even more doubtful of themselves. In fact, telling someone who is struggling that it is perfectly okay to have negative thoughts or to feel low can be more helpful than positive affirmations. On the other hand, affirmations can be helpful when we are seeking to reframe our internal dialogues—which can have a big impact on how we show up in the world, given that so many of us are plagued by feelings of inadequacy. Affirmations can be particularly powerful when they are contextual and backed by action.

Given that we are all bombarded with so many images on every social media platform every day, we are consuming way too much information and are continuously affected by external factors. The only way to protect yourself from all this is to actively cultivate some stillness in your day. It could be staying away from your phone for a few hours, going for a long walk, practicing some form of meditation or just sitting idle for some time doing nothing. John Lennon said, 'The time you enjoyed wasting is not wasted time'. There is a lot that happens in our brains when we are still, allowing us to get back in touch with ourselves and start to build the narrative of who we are and what truly matters to us, as opposed to being continually affected by some ideal image out there.

MENTAL HEALTH IN THE AGE OF ISOLATION

They say no man is an island, but the COVID-19 pandemic that raged across the world, profoundly altering the way we live, work and communicate, left huge numbers of people feeling more alone than ever. The idea of loneliness as a trigger for poor health—both physical and mental—is not new, but it has come into the spotlight as people grow more isolated, working from home, unable to visit loved ones or connect in person with their communities. Fear of the virus has led to increased social anxiety and generalized anxiety, but even those without a mental health diagnosis are struggling with feelings of loneliness.

Humans are social animals, even if some of us might consider ourselves introverts. We thrive on connection, and our brains and bodies are just happier when we experience social contact. Studies have found that loneliness is linked to increased risk for high blood pressure, heart disease, obesity, as well as depression and cognitive decline.[4] While most studies addressing the effects of isolation on health focused on older adults, research since the pandemic has looked at adults of all ages. One study found that the negative impact of social isolation was experienced even by young adults during COVID-19-related lockdowns. They reported lower levels of life satisfaction and overall wellness, experienced higher levels of work-related stress, and turned to unhealthy coping mechanisms including substance use.[5]

In addition to loneliness, the pandemic caused grief due to the loss of loved ones, financial stress due to the loss of jobs, and an atmosphere of uncertainty and fear. All of this has increased the risk for and incidence of many mental health disorders including panic, anxiety, depression, obsessive-compulsive disorders and post-traumatic stress.[6]

Many believe that loneliness will be the next global pandemic that we will have to grapple with. With couples choosing to marry later, and to have children later—or not at all—people were already facing new forms of social isolation. However, this has been exacerbated by the coronavirus and its fallout. In fact, recognizing the dangers of rising loneliness, Japan appointed a Minister for Loneliness in February 2021.[7] The minister's mandate is to attempt to tackle the rising rates of suicide in the country, especially among women who are hit particularly hard by the effects of social isolation. Initiatives like this, at a policy level, will hopefully address the issue before it reaches the levels of a pandemic.

In addition to our evolving lifestyles and family relationships, social media has also played a role in feelings of isolation. Spending hours scrolling through timelines, comparing ourselves and our lives to the glittering lives of influencers and celebrities, all while living in a time of instant gratification, contribute to feelings of loneliness.

In some Western countries, new age start-ups are emerging that facilitate interaction among younger people looking to earn some income and older people who are dealing with isolation. These companies connect the two and facilitate regular paid engagements where the person shows up to just be around, helping with chores, going for a walk or just having a chat. Some companies are even experimenting with a model in which the younger people accumulate social points, which they can similarly encash for company when they reach old age.

HEALTH HACK #23: Find Gratitude

Pausing every now and then to feel grateful and give thanks can actually make you feel healthier, whether you practice gratitude meditation or maintain a gratitude journal. Even the simple act of calling someone who has made a difference in your life and thanking them for being there for you can significantly improve your feelings of wellbeing.

SEEKING MENTAL WELLNESS

In many ways, to be human is to feel things—grief, worry, anger, irritability, as well as joy, pride, excitement and anticipation. Some amount of stress and anxiety, unfortunately, are also inescapable in the world we now live in. The incredibly powerful brains that evolution has blessed us with allow us to think complex and wonderful thoughts, but also make it possible for us to overthink, worry about the future and analyse everything to the point of distraction. It is important to seek help whenever you feel your thoughts or emotions are coming in the way of your normal function—affecting your work, your relationships, or your general state of mind. The common advice is to seek help if you have trouble sleeping, changes in appetite, an inability to concentrate or perform daily functions and a loss of enjoyment in fun activities. Particularly if you have been struggling with any of these for six weeks or more, it is likely that an intervention can help you and it would be best to speak to a professional. Some people, however, believe that therapy is for everybody, and not simply for those experiencing a period of struggle. In fact, speaking to a therapist even when you don't feel unwell, can help build resilience and give you the tools you need to face harder times.

Unlike most other physical illnesses which require rest or medication, mental illnesses are unique in that we might benefit from talking to another person, especially if that person is a professional who knows how to listen, what to focus on and how to drive the patient's attention to modes of thinking that can make the management of the condition better. Over the last one hundred years, many therapy techniques have been developed which are all effective in different contexts. Most forms of therapy help us get in touch with ourselves, identifying childhood traumas or relationships that might have had a profound impact on us before we were even aware of it. They might help us develop better self-awareness or offer tools that enable us to control our response to situations.

One of the most researched forms of therapy is Cognitive Behavioural Therapy (CBT), in which the job of the therapist is to help the patient see that they are separate from their thoughts and that, with some practice, they can learn to let their thoughts come and go without affecting them. CBT raises patient awareness over a period and equips them with mental techniques to deal with tricky situations as they arise. Counselling is a very widespread form of therapy that mostly comprises active listening and guiding the patient to talk it out in a safe and non-judgemental environment. If you have ever felt better after unloading your frustration to a sympathetic listener, you know how counselling works. It is particularly effective with mild and short-term issues.

Counsellors can empathetically listen and nudge the patient towards specific patterns of thinking that lead to clearing the mind of unresolved thoughts.

There are several more options for therapy, including family or couples therapy, as well as art therapy that uses creative expression as an outlet for emotions. Every single one of us might benefit from not just a different style of therapy, but also a different therapist. It might take you a few tries to find the perfect person for you, but I would say hang in there, because it is ultimately worth it. Some people find that making that deep connection with a therapist is, in fact, more important than the therapist's credentials or the form of therapy they practice.

Advances in the field of medicine mean that there are now numerous drugs that have been found to be effective in treating mental health illnesses. Most of these work by targeting specific neurotransmitters and pathways to alter the underlying neurobiology, but since they directly affect the brain, addiction can be a threat. However, when prescribed by a psychiatrist and used in conjunction with therapy and other interventions, they might enable people living with mental illnesses to function better. In some cases, the medication can also be phased out once symptoms improve.

Some of the most common types of antidepressant medications are known as SSRIs (selective serotonin reuptake inhibitors) and, more recently, SNRIs (serotonin and norepinephrine reuptake inhibitors). Both these classes of medication do just what their names indicate i.e., block the reabsorption of the specific neurotransmitters, thus increasing their levels. Another class of drugs is anti-anxiety medication, which provides immediate relief from anxiety or panic and calms down the activity of the brain. Some of these work by boosting the presence of GABA transmitters whose depletion leads to feelings of anxiety and panic. All these drugs must be prescribed by a psychiatrist and the schedule of medication followed closely, with regular check-ins with your doctor.

We now have mountains of data on the positive impact of a healthy lifestyle on mental health. This is thanks to the intimate and powerful connection between the mind and the body. The modern movement towards integrative medicine very actively incorporates lifestyle changes. Whether it is about getting high quality sleep, going for a morning walk, engaging in activities that challenge the mind, incorporating meditation, working out regularly or eating brain boosting food, you are more likely to benefit from any mental health treatment if you approach it holistically. While medications provide much needed symptomatic relief and therapy unravels the deeper issues at play, a strong lifestyle protocol will create a healthy environment for your mind and body to flourish and restore balance that will help you get better in the long run as well.

As I've said before, there is no one-size-fits-all when it comes to mental health, and it might even require some trial and error, whether you try therapy, medication and lifestyle changes. This is why it is so important to work closely with a psychiatrist or trained therapist to find what works best for you. While there is no question that lifestyle plays an important role in how mental health issues develop and progress, there is also no mistaking a strong medical component as well. Mental health issues can range from very mild to being absolutely debilitating. The actual treatment protocol can only be designed by a trained professional, but there are several small steps you can take as preventive measures, to reduce the likelihood of developing mental health illness. Here are a few lifestyle interventions that are positively correlated with a significant reduction in occurrence and intensity.

1. Exercise: even if it is a walk or some gentle yoga. Movement can boost your mood, and I find that it helps to bust stress and alleviate anxiety.

2. Watch what you eat: to see if different kinds of foods make you feel differently. I've noticed that very heavy meals leave me feeling lethargic and unmotivated, while fasting and fibre rich meals give me the energy I need for the day.

3. Meditate: by choosing from a variety of techniques and using a guided meditation app if that works for you. Studies have proven that meditation in the long term can improve brain health. I find that even a few minutes of quiet contemplation can improve my focus.

4. Breathe: whether it is just taking a few deep breaths or practicing pranayama. Breathing techniques have become a very useful tool for me on particularly rough days, and now I know that science validates this.

5. Talk: to your family, friends, co-workers and to a therapist. Opening up about your emotions and experiences can lead to moments of profound connection and help you sort through your thoughts.

6. Test your blood sugar: studies have found links between blood glucose levels and mental health. For example, people with diabetes are more likely to have depression. Keeping an eye on your sugar might be a good idea if you've been struggling.

7. Supplement: ask your doctor or nutritionist if there are supplements, such as Omega-3 fatty acids, that could help with brain health and mental wellness.

8. Sleep: create rituals around bedtime that can help you get at least eight hours of rest every night.

Most importantly, don't worry if none of the above work for you. Speak to your doctors and therapists and try different things to see what makes you feel well, and don't lose hope. We live in a time where our understanding of mental health ailments is better than ever before and we have access to therapists and psychiatrists even in small towns now. There are excellent books and tons of online resources that you can use to build a deeper understanding to treat and manage your mental health just like you would with any other health issue.

Being There for Others

Seeking help for yourself is one part of the journey, but the other is being there for the people you love, who are struggling with their mental health. Being a caregiver, a partner, a relative or a friend to someone who is battling depression, anxiety or any other illness, can be a difficult role to play. It can be overwhelming and confusing when you don't know what to say or how to behave when someone you care about is going through a mental health crisis. This, in turn, can lead to more stress, affecting your ability to be there and support your loved one.

These are some of the things I have found to be the most useful:

- Listen: We often underestimate the importance of just listening, attentively, with care, and without any judgement or reaction. Communicating that you hear them and understand them can go a long way in creating a safe environment for a nurturing conversation.
- Understand: If there is a diagnosis, try to learn as much about it as you can. Use open-ended questions to gently help them open up to you.

- Be honest: Admit to your friend or relative if you're not sure what they need and ask how you can better support them.
- Remember the little things: Sometimes, small and thoughtful actions like a home-cooked meal or an invitation to go for a walk together can make all the difference and show someone how much you care. It's okay to occasionally distract your loved one from the source of their distress, giving them some relief.
- Be realistic about recovery: The journey of healing can be a long one and does not always follow a logical path. Being realistic about your expectations of recovery can help you manage your own responses to your loved one's distress.
- Ask for help: If you're ever worried about the person's safety or wellbeing, get in touch with a mental health professional immediately. Make sure to look after your own mental health in the process, so that their burdens don't become your own.

MENTAL HEALTH IN INDIA

In India, according to a 2016 report[8], 13.7 per cent of the population lives with mental health illnesses requiring an intervention. In addition, mood disorders and neurotic or stress-related disorders were two to three times more prevalent in urban than in rural areas. The most commonly occurring disorders were found to be depression, anxiety and substance abuse, which affect nearly ten per cent of the population. One in twenty Indians were living with depression, and depression was found to be higher in women aged between forty and forty-nine years, living in urban areas. The report also discovered that mental health illnesses were increasingly found in children and young adults, and that 9.5

million young Indians aged between thirteen and seventeen years required active intervention.

Despite increasing awareness of the importance of mental health, it remains an issue surrounded by preconceived notions, prejudice and shame. In addition, in India, the treatment gap, between the prevalence of mental health illness and the percentage of patients that receive treatment, is over 60 per cent.

The fact that so many people not only live with mental illnesses, but also live undiagnosed or untreated, means that the impact is immense. It affects the day-to-day functioning of patients, causing debilitating symptoms that prevent them from being able to live and work. As a result, the economic and social burden on individuals and families is also immense. Unfortunately, in India, mental health disorders are still associated with a great deal of stigma, and this might be one of the reasons so many are unable to seek the help they need.

On a more positive note however, there are more and more non-profit organizations and experts who are working tirelessly to increase awareness and reduce stigma. There is hope that the young people of today will have a better understanding of their mental health than any generation before them, transforming this field of health.

In Summary

Keep in Mind

1. Despite all the advances in medical sciences, mental health, which is crucial to overall health and wellness, continues to be shrouded in stigma.
2. Mental health is extraordinarily complex, difficult to diagnose, understand and treat.
3. Many experts in the field believe that we need to reframe our approach to mental health, not seeing them as moral deficiencies but as aspects of health that might need attention like any other.
4. Metacognition is the unique human ability to be aware of the self, thinking about our own thinking, and we can harness this self-awareness to recognize when we are falling into negative patterns or traps of emotional reactions.
5. While some stress is good for the health of our minds and bodies, much of the chronic stress we now experience takes a toll on our mental health.
6. Low levels of anxiety might help draw attention to a threat, but when it becomes chronic, it can negatively impact our daily function.
7. Depression is also considered a lifestyle disease and is a result of an imbalance of neurotransmitters, combined with lifestyle, genetic and environmental factors.
8. Trauma lies at the heart of many mental health challenges and working through them with an experienced therapist can help us unblock our minds and move forward.
9. Wellness culture through social media sometimes promotes toxic positivity, promoting the idea that anything less than happy perfection is inadequate.

10. Loneliness might be the next epidemic we face, as we grow increasingly isolated from friends and family in our modern world.

11. Various forms of therapy and medication can help manage mental health conditions, while lifestyle factors like exercise, better sleep and meditation can play a role in prevention.

Take Action

1. Pay attention to your sleep and fitness. Both can help immensely with boosting mood and providing resilience to deal with mental health.

2. Use guided meditation to increase self-awareness that can help you identify patterns of thought that lead you down a spiral of negativity or anxiety.

3. Make sure to manage your stress—through yoga, meditation, time in nature, or social activities—to make sure it does not have adverse effects on your mental health.

4. Speaking to a therapist, even if you do not have a mental health diagnosis, can be extraordinarily eye-opening, helping you unpack trauma you might never know you had.

5. If you find yourself feeling inadequate or depressed after spending time on your social media feeds, consider taking a break or following people who don't make you feel bad for not being 'happy' or 'perfect'.

6. Cultivate an active social network of trusted friends and family members who can provide you with a safe environment to discuss anything on your mind.

7. Spend time outdoors and in nature. Sunlight, trees, the sky and the ocean have a way of lifting our spirits.

8. If you keep facing the same issue again or you feel your energy sagging for no apparent reason, reach out to a mental health expert.

9. Be cognizant of people around you who might be dealing with mental health challenges. Approach them without judgement and extend whatever support you can, to help them deal with the situation.

PART 4

THE FUTURE

10

AGEING & LONGEVITY

Do not go gentle into that good night,
Old age should burn and rave at close of day;
Rage, rage against the dying of the light.

. . .

Grave men, near death, who see with blinding sight
Blind eyes could blaze like meteors and be gay,
Rage, rage against the dying of the light.

—Dylan Thomas

For as long as I remember, I've had an active lifestyle—a choice I made almost subconsciously. In fact, I hadn't put much thought into the implications of pursuing a healthy lifestyle, until 2006, when I read a book that changed my mindset forever. I picked up Ray Kurzweil's book, *Fantastic Voyage: Live Long Enough to Live Forever*, out of casual curiosity, little knowing that it would profoundly alter my perception of the human lifespan and the idea of ageing. I knew Kurzweil as a well-respected scientist and inventor with a phenomenal track record, but reading his book was truly an eye-opening moment for me.

I was deeply struck by the idea that ageing could be viewed as a disease—one that many leading scientists in the field of longevity research were working to cure. The possibility of a dramatic extension in the human lifespan piqued my interest, and from that moment on, I began to follow the exciting developments in the field. When I first heard of Human Longevity Inc, co-founded by one of the leaders of the first human genome draft sequencing project, I was excited by the enormous potential being unlocked by global organizations.

In 2015, I had the opportunity to visit the Human Longevity Inc (HLI) centre in San Diego, something I had only dreamt of. Through their platform 'Health Nucleus', they offer personalized and comprehensive healthcare, and I signed up for a day of rigorous testing. I arrived at the ultramodern, glass fronted building that houses Health Nucleus, as well as its parent company, HLI, situated on a sunny campus lined with palm trees. After being welcomed into a beautifully lit reception—not unlike that of a luxury spa—I was escorted to my personal suite, where I was given a set of soft cotton clothes and socks to wear for the day. I had to keep reminding myself that I hadn't just checked into a beach resort! After my vitals were measured, I had my blood drawn, followed by a consultation with a doctor about my health history. Each room I was guided into seemed more high-tech than the next, and the experience had a touch of the futuristic.

While my samples were drawn for full genome and microbiome sequencing, I spent almost an hour and a half doing a full body MRI. Fortunately, I got to choose music and visuals to keep me calm and relaxed as I lay inside the giant machine. After a few more scans and tests, I was done for the day, and checked out of the Health Nucleus clinic. The process offered me an extraordinarily detailed picture of what exactly was going on in my body at that point of time. In addition, I was able to get an incredible insight into my risk for certain illnesses, and what I could do to minimize that risk. To have a dashboard of sorts for your body has profound implications for your life and your health choices, making the sort of testing done by HLI a truly powerful exercise.

At the time I visited the Health Nucleus, it was an expensive proposition. Now, however, much of this technology—while still cutting-edge—has become a lot more affordable. For example, you can get your genome and microbiome sequenced for around Rs 10,000/-, a number that is still coming down. What was on the fringe just five or six years ago is now coming into the mainstream. Longevity has started to become a solution that companies are offering, and it really is an exciting time to be alive.

It is said that the day we are born, we begin to die. This might sound like a somewhat pessimistic outlook on life, but the truth is that ageing and eventual death from old age have always been viewed as inevitable. So deeply entrenched is our fear of this unavoidable fate, that old age has often been considered a time of weakness, powerlessness and vulnerability, even in mythology. *Geras* is the personification of old age in the Greek myths, and he was a frail, shrivelled up old man. From Homeric Hymn 5[1] to Aphrodite, these lines reveal the suspicion, fear and hatred of old age: 'Harsh old age (*Geras*) will soon enshroud you—ruthless age which stands someday at the side of every man, deadly, wearying, dreaded even by the gods.'

The modern theories of ageing have presented us with a revolutionary new idea—that ageing is not inevitable. It is becoming increasingly clear that the decline and disease that accompany old age can be postponed, avoided and perhaps even reversed. And instead, we can enjoy energy, good health and vigour, well into our later years. It's also important to acknowledge the positive side of ageing. It is believed that due to the deactivation of the amygdala, old people experience less fear, while discovering an emotional balance.[2] A big part of how we age depends on genetics, environment, personality and even how we view ageing itself.

In almost every culture of the world, the wisdom of the elderly is considered a constant. Think of the many folk tales and myths that feature a wise old woman or a knowledgeable grandfather figure. To what does age owe its wisdom? Studies have found that as people age, they become better at pattern recognition and abstraction. They might forget many of the minor details of everyday life, like where they left the TV remote or their neighbour's name, but they are more likely to have a better sense of the 'bigger picture'. This could be because they have a wealth of experience to turn back to, and neural pathways forged by those experiences. However, having certain neural connections ingrained in their brains does not mean that older people are too set in their ways to learn something new. The brain is incredibly malleable, even in later years. Just look at Colonel Sanders who founded KFC at the age of sixty-two! Or the artist Anna Mary Robertson Moses, often referred to as Grandma Moses, who started painting at the age of seventy-eight and went on to have her works displayed at New York's Museum of Modern Art.

While ageing and death are very much a part of human life, we are now in a position to craft a plan to considerably slow down the process and reduce the chances of developing the debilitating diseases of old age that are often taken for granted.

If we can find a way of thriving even in old age, the possibilities become endless.

From birth to early adulthood, our bodies just keep growing in leaps and bounds, as if powered by a magic potion. We get bigger, stronger, smarter; we have bright, youthful skin; we recover rapidly from infections and injuries; and, barring a few hormone fuelled and moody teenage years, we are filled with a sense of adventure and unbridled enthusiasm. We boast of incredible metabolism that allows us to eat practically anything without gaining weight. We can party into the early hours of the morning and still show up for work, bursting with energy. We feel invincible.

It seems like nothing can go wrong until it inevitably does, gradually, first in our late twenties and accelerating through our thirties and forties. This is the age at which most people start to gain weight, men begin to lose their hair and everyone's skin starts to look worn out. There are days when we wonder whether we will have the energy to get out of bed, let alone get through the day. The body continues its inevitable march towards older age, often accompanied by the onset of lifestyle diseases in the forties, which get exacerbated in the fifties and sixties.

Depending on how your middle years went, you may look like a mere shadow of your youthful self, relying on an army of doctors and innumerable pills just to get through the days and nights. Fortunately, however, there has been intense research into how our bodies age, and what we can do to slow the decline while dramatically increasing health span—to ensure that we can live with vitality and health well into older age. In fact, thanks to science, we no longer have to accept declining health as the only way to age, thus changing the way in which we perceive the very idea of ageing.

HEALTH HACK #24: Exercise the Brain

The brain needs a workout as much as our biceps do. Anything that engages and challenges the faculties of the mind can help boost its performance, including Sudoku and crossword puzzles, meditation sessions and brain game apps like Lumosity or Peak.

THE SCIENCE OF AGEING

Why we age has been one of the great mysteries of our lives. It seems as though our bodies are programmed to cycle from the vigour of youth to the gradual decline of old age, until the frail body withers away. And yet, until very recently, we knew little about what caused this process. There have been many theories, however, and the picture is becoming clearer with the rapid progress in the science of ageing. One of the first clues to ageing came from what's known as the Hayflick Limit which refers to the number of times a cell can divide before cell death occurs. Normal human cells can divide a maximum of forty to sixty times, and these divisions also affect telomere length. As cells divide, chance mutations occur, damaging the efficacy of the DNA and leading to many compromises in cell function.

Other clues come from flora and fauna in the wild. Bowhead whales are known to live for over two hundred years, while bristlecone pine trees live for up to 5,000 years! This fact inspired scientists to look for 'longevity genes', which protect the body and appeared to be turned on by adversity. These scientists then began to study yeast cells, flies and other model organisms to identify these particular genes and pathways that seemed to slow down the ageing process.

One of the most common theories of ageing is based on the idea of free radical damage. Just in case you need a quick refresher, free radicals are molecules of oxygen that have split into single atoms, leaving unpaired electrons scavenging the body for other electrons. The result is oxidative stress, which has been compared to the rusting of the body, damaging cells, proteins and DNA. Ageing has often been linked to the gradual build-up of free radical damage in the body, which is believed to be one of the causes of many age-related disorders, from Alzheimer's to cancer. Antioxidants are often depicted as the cure-all for oxidative stress, and they do mitigate the harmful effects of free radicals to some extent. However, their role in anti-ageing has probably been exaggerated. Regular exercise and certain dietary sources—including a variety of colourful fruits and vegetables, some kinds of tea and the compounds in red wine—can give your body the required amounts of antioxidants to fight the damage of free radicals. However, free radical damage is not the biggest factor in the ageing process until late in life, and, even then, is found to be reversible.

While researchers and scientists around the world have been unable to reach a consensus on a single theory of ageing, there has been some agreement that certain hallmarks of ageing seem to exist. In his book, *Ageless: The New Science of Getting Older Without Getting Old*, biologist Andrew Steele defines these hallmarks as factors that either accumulate with age, factors whose presence accelerates the ageing process, or factors that, when removed, improve the situation. They are as follows:

1. Unstable genes as a result of DNA damage
2. Shortening of telomeres, the protective caps at the ends of chromosomes

3. Epigenomic changes which determine which genes are turned on or off
4. Loss of healthy proteostasis or the maintenance of protein
5. Deregulated nutrient sensing or a lowered ability of cells to identify and respond to nutrients
6. Mitochondrial dysfunction
7. Accumulation of senescent zombie-like cells that cause inflammation
8. Lowered or empty reserves of stem cells
9. Changes in communication between cells and the production of inflammatory molecules
10. Early research suggests that loss of diversity in the microbiome could cause age-related inflammation
11. Decline in the functioning of the immune system due to the loss of cells in the thymus where T-cells originate

The idea, then, is to address these hallmarks, in order to address or slow down ageing and its related diseases.

Scientists have identified three 'longevity genes' or pathways that can be exploited to slow down, or even reverse, the ageing process. The 'mTOR', or the mammalian target of rapamycin, is a longevity gene that makes a protein, which senses the presence of amino acids in the body, using this as a signal to build muscles, for example after a protein-rich meal. Studies have found that downregulated mTOR activity leads to a longer life, as the body hunkers down into survival mode. Instead of building new proteins, a process called autophagy, which recycles proteins, seems to be better for longevity. Lab mice who are given rapamycin, a drug given as an immunosuppressant that inhibits mTOR activity, live much longer lives.

AMPK is a pathway that is turned on in response to low levels of energy in the body, such as during fasted states. When activated, AMPK increases glucose sensitivity and boosts the production of mitochondria, the energy houses of the cell. This pathway has also been found to be linked to increased longevity. Metformin, considered one of the safest drugs that has been used as the major treatment of type 2 diabetes, is found to activate AMPK. Studies have found that patients of diabetes, who have been on metformin, tend to live longer than people who don't even have diabetes. Research is now being conducted into the specific effects of metformin on longevity. In response to low energy, AMPK also downregulates mTOR and activates other longevity genes.

The third longevity pathway is a family of genes known as sirtuins. While studying yeast cells in his lab, biologist David Sinclair and his team discovered a gene mutation known as silent information regulator-2 or SIR2, that was associated with longevity. Studies have since found the same family of genes in humans, which are activated by fasting and by exercise, and associated with longevity.

All three of these longevity genes respond to biological stress, altering genes so that cells hunker down to survive a period of difficulty, while boosting DNA repair and mitochondrial function or reducing inflammation. Therefore, some amount of stress—that does not end in cell damage—is good for us (remember the concept of hormesis), including certain kinds of exercise, exposure to extreme temperatures or caloric restriction as in intermittent fasting.

Some of the ways to boost sirtuin and AMPK activity while inhibiting the mTOR pathway—all of which are now thought to boost longevity by addressing the various hallmarks of ageing—include caloric restriction or periods of fasting, exercise, immersion in cold temperatures, as well as certain medicines that mimic these forms of hormesis, including supplements like metformin, rapamycin and resveratrol. By now it shouldn't come as a surprise to you that exercise and caloric restriction are routes to living not just healthier, but also longer, lives.

AGEING IN THE GENES

An understanding of what goes on inside our genes as we age can help us better grasp the modern theories of ageing. As you might already know, each of our cells has a nucleus that contains all its genetic information. Inside the nucleus of every cell, long strands of DNA are wrapped around proteins called histones, which form chromosomes. Every type of cell, from those of the brain to those of the liver or the heart or the skin, has its DNA packaged or wrapped in a very specific way that defines what kind of cell it will be. Cells inherit this information about what type of cell they need to be through epigenetics, which controls which genes are more tightly wrapped and which are readable or 'turned on'.

With age, cells seem to lose their identity through what David Sinclair describes as the unravelling of DNA. Thus confused, cells lose their specificity, becoming more generalized and unable to function as they were meant to. Sinclair believes that this process, known as ex-differentiation, lies at the root of ageing and all its associated diseases. For example, this happens to the neurons or the cells of the brain in the case of Alzheimer's Disease—they forget what exactly they are meant to do, resulting in problems of memory and cognition. This is also what happens in type 2 diabetes, when cells in the lining of blood vessels lose their ability to absorb the glucose from the bloodstream—achieved through a gene known as GLUT-4. It is interesting to note that two such different diseases, as well as several others, including heart disease, might be caused by the same thing—ex-differentiation.

Sinclair, as well as other scientists working at the cutting edge of ageing, thus believe that we can address these diseases by fixing the epigenetic disruptions in the cells of our body and essentially reversing ageing. Instead of focusing on individual therapies or drugs for each type of disease, their intention is to focus on the longevity genes and pathways to reset our biological clocks.

Speaking of biological clocks, there are now techniques of measuring one's biological age. While anyone who knows their date of birth knows their chronological age, the number of years we have existed on the face of the earth is not always an accurate measure of our body's true age. In 2013, geneticist and biostatistician Steve Horvath published a paper which showed that the bundling or unravelling of DNA, patterns known as DNA methylation, could be measured to gauge biological age. This came to be known as the Horvath clock, which is based on epigenetics, as DNA methylation can switch genes on or off. DNA methylation is a linear process that changes with age, but lifestyle and environmental stressors can speed up or alter the process.

With technology advancing rapidly and becoming more affordable, it might soon be possible for every single one of us to understand not only our biological ages, but also find out when we will die. As frightening as this sounds, there is comfort in the fact that the scientists working on these technologies also believe that biological ageing can be slowed and even reversed, helping us extend both our lifespans and our health spans.

While the theories of ageing are evolving as science pushes the boundaries of the unknown, it seems as though good health and even longevity come down to better lifestyles—once again cutting-edge modern research confirms what our ancestors already knew.

Genes & DNA

A quick look at how far the study of genetics has come can help us understand just how advanced the science of longevity now is.

James Watson and Francis Crick unleashed the genetic genie on the world of medicine in 1953 with their discovery of the double helix structure of the DNA molecule. DNA is the fundamental building block of the human body which contains the code to build life from scratch. Every single cell of our body contains a fully intact DNA molecule, which makes it theoretically possible to create a clone from just a single cell. A single DNA molecule is made of about three billion base pairs, each of which can be thought of as a single letter—A, T, C and G. Specific long stretches of these four letters in a particular sequence are known as genes, combinations that encode chemical instructions for building various proteins and enzymes in the right environment.

Humans possess about 20,000 genes and these orchestrate everything that happens from birth to death. And yet, it isn't quite so simple. As much as we'd all like to believe the sensational news headlines about scientists discovering a 'gene for obesity' or a 'gene for longevity', the truth is far more complex. Far from having a single gene for every trait, there are usually dozens and often hundreds involved in executing a particular function.

One of the most fiercely debated subjects in the field of science and biology has been about what makes us who we are. This nature–nurture argument questions whether it is our genes or the environment in which we are raised that exerts the greatest influence on our development and personalities. The study of epigenetics has finally begun to shed light on this eternal debate, and it appears that the way genes express themselves can vary dramatically, depending on the environment they are in. This environment includes the environment inside the womb before birth, as well as early childhood and social environment, and could also include learned behaviours and lifestyle. Some of the most powerful illustrations of this interaction between nature and nurture come from studies on identical twins who were separated at birth. It has been found that certain traits, like eye colour for example, seem to be solely determined by genetics, while most characteristics, including personality and personal preferences, are a result of a complex interplay of genes and the environment.

While debate on the specifics of how much we draw on our genes and our environment rages on, the fact itself is excellent news for managing our health. To know that we are not at the mercy of the genetic lottery, but that we can influence the way our genes manifest themselves by making conscious choices, is hugely empowering. For example, while diabetes and obesity might be genetically inherited, one's environment and lifestyle will also determine whether they are expressed. As many scientists now say, 'Your genes are not your destiny'.

With the impressive strides made by scientists in the study of genetics, it became possible to predict certain diseases by identifying specific problems in the functioning of specific genes. By the 1960s, doctors could even diagnose some disorders in babies while they were still in the womb, such as Down Syndrome, in which babies are born with a duplicate copy of chromosome 21.

By the 1990s, geneticists had mapped most Mendelian disorders, which are inherited diseases caused by a defect in a single gene. However, in order to understand how genes affected the more complex illnesses, we needed a clearer and more complete understanding of our genes. Thus, the Human Genome Project was launched in 1990 as a vast, global and collaborative study with the ambitious goal of accurately sequencing and mapping the entire human genome, which is made up of three billion DNA base pairs. The project was completed in 2003, opening up a world of insight into the human species.

While the first complete sequence of the human genome took over ten years and cost billions of dollars, the cost of sequencing has been falling dramatically in recent times. Now, you can do a basic genetic test for less than 10,000 rupees and a full genetic sequencing for just 50,000 rupees. It is incredibly cool to know that we can read the codebook of our own lives—letter by letter, understanding what it means for our health. For example, a genetic test might help us discover a susceptibility to certain inheritable diseases, allowing us to take action accordingly. It could also tell us what kind of food and exercise are more amenable to our unique genetic constitutions and what deficiencies we can proactively address. With the increasing knowledge of how genes function, we will soon have customized therapies and treatments tailored for our unique bodies and problems.

One area, in which gene sequencing is already having a dramatic effect, is the treatment of cancers. Cancers are sometimes caused by genetic mutations that lead cells to divide in an uncontrolled manner, eventually hijacking many of the body's functions. Using sequencing techniques, oncologists can now identify the exact mutation in a patient and then create a personalized drugs plan to target that mutation. As a result of such advanced technologies, the recovery rates for cancers have improved significantly.

Telomeres

One of the hallmarks of ageing, telomeres have been likened to the plastic ends of shoelaces and called the goalkeepers of a cell. As illustrated by the shoelace metaphor, they are repetitive

DNA sequences located at the ends of chromosomes that protect cells from degeneration. However, telomeres shorten with cell replication, and it is believed that when they are shortened beyond a point, the cell becomes senescent or stops replication, leading to ageing.

By protecting chromosomes, telomeres maintain genomic integrity, but their shortening leads to instability in genes. Telomere length is maintained by an enzyme called telomerase, which can add telomeres to the ends of chromosomes that have been worn down, thus slowing down or reversing their shortening with age. With the discovery of telomeres and telomerase, scientists also realized that we can control the ageing process to some degree by looking after our telomeres. Techniques that address the mind and the body, like meditation and Qigong, reduce stress and increase telomerase. Cardiovascular exercise and a diet of healthy, whole foods are also found to improve telomere health.

Since the discovery of telomeres, there has been exciting research not only into their role in ageing, but also their relationship with stress. Elissa Epel and Elizabeth Blackburn, who have done cutting-edge research in the field, found that the mothers of children with chronic conditions, who had high levels of perceived stress, had shorter telomeres and lower levels of telomerase, compared to mothers of healthy children.[3] In both groups, mothers with higher levels of perceived stress had less healthy telomeres. This study proved that cellular ageing could be affected by our lifestyles and our responses to stress. Studies have found that anxiety and depression are also linked to shorter telomeres, while meditation and exercise can help boost their health.[4]

In addition, fitness levels also impact telomere length, as one study of 1,200 pairs of identical twins found—the twin who exercised and stayed active was found to have longer telomeres than the less active twin.[5] There are some kinds of exercise that are better for our telomeres than others—moderate aerobic endurance and high intensity interval training. However, increasing any kind of activity can lead to an increase in telomerase levels.

Telomere length is negatively affected by too much exercise, too little or poor quality sleep, lifestyle diseases like diabetes, diets rich in refined carbohydrates and sugars, high stress levels and lives that are low in social connections. In addition, one's environment also plays a role in determining telomere health, including aspects such as pollution, access to green spaces, dust and cigarette smoke.

Perhaps more significant than the possibility of being able to supplement telomerase, however, is the idea that the health of our telomeres lies, to a great extent, in our hands. Like many other elements of our health, it was assumed that genetics was the sole factor that determined the length of our telomeres, but we now know that the lifestyle choices we make play a role as important, if not more. In fact, it isn't just our lifestyle choices but also our mindset and attitudes that determine the length of our telomeres.

THE ROLE OF MITOCHONDRIA

You might remember mitochondria from your high school biology textbook, as the 'powerhouse of the cell'. However, it's likely that you don't remember much else about it because it only featured in passing. Recent research, however, has revealed that our mitochondria might play a far more significant role than we thought in almost every aspect of health, from cancer to Alzheimer's, while also being one of the hallmarks of ageing.

Mitochondria are organelles within our cells that, according to one hypothesis, were once separate bacteria-like organisms that were eventually enveloped by our cells in a uniquely endosymbiotic relationship. Every cell in our body has between a few hundred and a couple of thousand mitochondria within it. The cells of organs and tissues that require significant amounts of energy to function, such as the heart, brain or skeletal muscles, have greater concentrations of mitochondria. A fun fact about mitochondria is that they have their own DNA, mtDNA, which is passed on maternally. Given this, we can trace our lineage back to a woman who walked the earth around 1,70,000 years ago, known more popularly as Mitochondrial Eve. Who would have thought that all of humanity might indeed share a common mother!

Mitochondria capture the oxygen we breathe in and, through a complex process that breaks down the glucose derived from the food we eat, bind the released energy into tiny storage units known as ATP. ATP is like a little battery that stores usable energy to be drawn on when the body needs it. Since energy drives everything we do, healthy mitochondrial function is critical for a healthy lifestyle.

Mitochondria are now known to play a role in homeostasis, in signalling pathways within cells, and in responding to stressors. Another crucial function that mitochondria serve is in apoptosis or cell 'suicide'. When mitochondria receive certain stimuli, they ensure the controlled death of a cell. You might be wondering why the death of a cell is considered a good thing, but just imagine a malignant cell in a tumour. If it did not receive a signal to kill itself, it would keep growing unchecked and result in cancer.

With age—as free radical damage accumulates—or due to mitochondrial disorders, the capacity of our cells to produce energy is diminished. And this lowered supply of energy, in turn, affects the functioning of our body's organs. For example, the cardiovascular system is almost entirely controlled by the smooth muscles of the autonomic system, and these muscles require a significant amount of ATP to function well. The brain makes up only 2 per cent of the body's weight and yet uses 20 per cent of its total energy, illustrating how dependent this organ is on proper mitochondrial function. In fact, any malfunction in these powerhouses can lead to a host of neurodegenerative disorders, from Parkinson's and Alzheimer's to Huntington's disease.

As the scientific world continues its research into mitochondria, it is discovering links between the health of our mitochondria and the functioning of almost all the major systems of our body. Abnormal functioning of the mitochondria is related to mood disorders such as depression, as well as ADHD. The visible signs of ageing on our skin—wrinkles, dullness, sagging—are thought to be caused by the weakened functioning of mitochondria in the fibroblasts: cells that produce collagen and elastin. Even our stem cells depend on the health of their mitochondria to continue their renewal. [6]

So, what can we do to maintain our mitochondria and reduce the production of damaging free radicals? Studies have found that many antibiotics and prescription drugs lead to disruptions in the functioning of mitochondria by impairing the production of ATP or increasing the release of free radicals. Statins, which are prescribed increasingly often to control cholesterol levels, are also known to lead to various kinds of mitochondrial dysfunction.

Exercise is crucial to maintain the health of your cells, and your mitochondria in particular. However, when it comes to mitochondrial function, it appears that there is such a thing as too much exercise. Overexertion and activity that is too strenuous, without time taken out for rest and recovery, can increase the release of free radicals. So, exercise in moderation is what the doctor orders for your mitochondria's sake. Protecting against toxins and pollutants in your environment will also protect your mitochondria. Mitochondria play such a crucial role in health and ageing, that taking care of these tiny powerhouses can positively impact longevity.

THE BLUE ZONES

One of the most fascinating health stories that has caught our collective imagination is that of the Blue Zones. These are pockets of the world that see a disproportionately high percentage of centenarians. Their existence has sparked the excitement of numerous teams of eager scientists, who want to decode the secret of a long and healthy life. The term was first used by French demographer Michel Poulain and Italian researcher Giovanni Mario Pes in 2000, when they observed an extraordinary number of centenarians on the Italian island of Sardinia, concentrated in the mountainous Barbagia region. At around the same time, writer and National Geographic fellow Dan Buettner began to travel across the Blue Zones to find the secrets of some of the world's longest living populations.[7]

There are five Blue Zones: the mountainous highlands of Sardinia in Italy, the remote island of Okinawa in Japan, the coastal town of Nicoya in Costa Rica, the Mormon town of Loma Linda in California and Ikaria, an island in Greece. These regions have been studied extensively, yielding insights into a few common lifestyle patterns that seem to be associated with longevity and health. Here are some of the key ideas that emerge from studies of the Blue Zones:

Movement

The residents of the Blue Zones are always on the move. Most of these areas are remote, with rough terrain, very low population densities and few options for transport other than walking. This is why it's rare to see people here idling away their time on rocking chairs or in front of TVs. This is as true of a young woman as of a ninety-year-old veteran who was an adult during the Second World War! Movement is just an essential part of their lives.

Community

Close-knit communities are a feature shared by all the Blue Zones; communities in which people are deeply involved in each other's lives, celebrating special occasions together and supporting one another through hard times. They rarely, if ever, feel alone, in contrast to city life, where many struggle with loneliness even living in buildings with hundreds of other residents. In the Blue Zones, neighbours and friends wander into each other's homes for a cup of tea or a glass of wine whenever they feel the need.

Moderation

Okinawans recite a poetic mantra before every meal. 'Hara hachi bu' is a reminder to stop eating when you are 80 per cent full.[8] Most Blue Zone cultures share this practice of minimalism and moderation in their diets and lifestyles, often eating only two meals a day and occasionally practicing some form of fasting. The centenarians of these regions would probably share a good laugh if they heard how modern, cutting-edge science has only just discovered the many benefits of caloric restriction—laughter that would perhaps add a few more years to their already long lives!

Downtime & Rejuvenation

Studies of the Blue Zones have found that some downtime during the day not only acts as an antidote to stress, but also helps instil a sense of meaning and purpose—which contribute to a long and healthy life. Ways of downshifting vary, from taking a daily afternoon nap, to finding purpose in prayer, or having one day of the week on which to spend time with family and take a complete break from work.

You might have noticed that, apart from the geographical terrain of the Blue Zones, every other feature, habit and behaviour of the longest living populations can quite easily be replicated anywhere in the world. While it might be tempting to find a single secret ingredient or miracle elixir for a long life, the truth is that it is actually a complex mix of nutrition, physical activity, social connection, purpose and more that leads to a long life of vitality.

HEALTH HACK #25: Stem Cell Therapy

Stem cell therapy is the use of stem cells in the treatment and prevention of disease and injury. While research is still underway, the field has the potential to transform many aspects of healthcare, from cancer treatment to regenerative medicine.

STEMMING COGNITIVE DECLINE

As crazy as it might sound, we can exercise the brain to keep it healthy and fit, just as we do the body. Both work on the 'use it or lose it' principle, which means that the more their parts are engaged in activities and exercises, the more they respond and strengthen. On the other hand, left idle, the brain, like the body, will wither away. The brain is vulnerable to the effects of an unhealthy lifestyle as well as to age-related damage, but we can delay or reverse this decline by staying mentally active and sharp.

Despite recent research proving adult neurogenesis—or the birth of new neurons in adults—many of us still believe that as we age, we are less able to learn new skills or study new fields. The fact is, however, that by stimulating our brains through learning, reflecting, performing cognitively challenging tasks and even doing psychotherapy, we can take better care of them in the long term.

It is never too late to pick up a new habit. The act of learning, struggling and getting better will not only add a cool trick to your repertoire, but it will also do wonders for the health of your brain. It doesn't matter if you learn a physically demanding skill (like yoga or hiking) or a more creative one (painting or poetry); any activity that gainfully engages your brain is good for you. You will need to form new mental models to understand the principles of the new activity, starting with the building blocks, and slowly combining the basics to master higher levels of performance. These will be embedded in newly formed neural connections in the brain, boosting and strengthening its health.

If you don't think you have the time to commit to learning something new, however, don't despair. Staying mentally active can include doing a crossword or Sudoku puzzle every day, brushing up on your language or maths skills, and even playing an instrument you might have learnt as a child. Challenging your brain with tougher activities and problems, as well as regularly changing up the kinds of activities you engage in, are all ways of stimulating the brain in holistic and effective ways.

The hippocampus is the part of the brain responsible for memory and learning, and is also particularly responsive to changes in neural circuitry and thus, to plasticity. According to Peter Hollins in his book *How to Build a Better Brain: Using Everyday Neuroscience to Train Your Brain for Motivation, Discipline, Courage and Mental Sharpness,* about 700 new brain cells are born in the hippocampus every day. The hippocampus also grows in response to physical exercise and can be protected or repaired by increasing the intake of foods high in Omega-3 fatty acids and avoiding alcohol.

In fact, studies have shown that it's not just general mental activity that best stimulates the brain but challenging ones that explore new areas and encourage the development of new neural connections. In a 2013 study at the University of Texas in Dallas, researchers randomly assigned 221 senior citizens between the ages of sixty and ninety to take up an activity, for about fifteen hours per week, over a period of three months.[9] One group took up learning a new skill—either digital photography or quilting—while the other group did more familiar activities like word puzzles, listening to music or socializing. After the three-month period, as well as a year after the study, those who had learnt a new skill scored far better on tests of memory than those who had engaged in other activities. And, interestingly, those who learnt digital photography fared better than those who learnt quilting, perhaps indicating that the more challenging and unfamiliar a skill was, the better effect it has on the brain.

Apart from exercising those brain cells, it's also important to protect them from the dangers of modern life. Chronic stress, which is ongoing but often goes unnoticed, can affect the structure of the brain. For example, studies have shown that it can cause a 14 per cent decrease in the volume of the hippocampus, thus impairing memory, processing and overall brain function. In addition to managing stress, it is important to get at least seven to eight hours of sleep every single night. With its role in memory and processing, sleep is like a tonic for the brain.

I find it utterly fascinating that we can actively cultivate better brain health and, in the process, not only improve our overall health but also the quality of our lives. Our brain responds to every type of stimulus—positive and negative—and grows in response to what we feed it. It is not only the most complex object in the whole universe, but also an absolutely malleable one. Taking control of one's mind and actively nurturing it can continue to pay dividends throughout life.

In Summary

Keep in Mind

1. We have always considered ageing to be an inevitable side effect of being human, but a new school of thought views ageing as a disease that can be treated and even reversed, expanding our lifespans and health spans.
2. While there is no single theory of ageing, it is believed to be related to a number of things, including and perhaps most importantly, a loss of definition in cells due to unravelling DNA. Scientists have identified three pathways or 'longevity genes' that can be harnessed to slow down or even reverse ageing.
3. Genes are not our destiny. Our lifestyle, environment and experience can influence the expression of our genes, giving us more control over our health than we imagined.
4. The shortening of telomeres—the protective end caps of chromosomes—has been linked to ageing, but lifestyle changes can slow down or even reverse this process.
5. The tiny mitochondria in our cells that power our bodies are closely linked to the health of every physiological function. Exercise and supplements can improve their function.
6. The ageing brain needs exercise and engagement, just as the ageing body does.

Take Action

1. Two simple ways for you to turn on your longevity genes, if you want to live longer and healthier, are to eat less and exercise more.

2. If you want to take your health to the next level, sign up for a basic genetic test, or even full genome sequencing. The results will help you better tailor your lifestyle to your unique genetic makeup.

3. Make sure to handle your stress—whether this involves meditating, spending time with family, or taking regular breaks and vacations—in order to take better care of your telomeres.

4. Moderate exercise can help you protect your mitochondria, as can keeping an eye on your exposure to toxins in the environment.

5. To live longer and better lives, the advice of some of the world's longest living communities is to move, stay connected to friends and family, eat less and take the time to rest, relax and rediscover a sense of purpose.

6. To slow down cognitive decline, keep your brain active: learn a new skill, do daily crosswords and word puzzles, brush up your maths or language skills.

11

BECOMING SUPERHUMAN

When I woke up this morning, one of the first things I did was to check out my Oura app on my phone to see how my health dashboard was looking. I'd received a sleep score of ninety and my readiness score was ninety-two—one of the best I've got so far. These numbers are a far cry from my scores from a year ago, when I first started wearing the Oura Ring—a nifty wearable health tracking device. A year ago, my scores were all in the sixties or seventies, and this was so demoralizing, that, at one point, I even stopped wearing the Oura Ring completely!

Eventually, I made my way back to wearing it, this time determined to figure out how to fix my scores, especially when it came to sleep. The Oura Ring, like other devices, offers useful insights into sleep in addition to tracking it quite accurately. I began to pay close attention to what seemed to affect the quality of my sleep, and I began to understand the correlation between the time of my last meal and the time I went to bed. When I ate dinner late in the evening and went to sleep soon after, my heart rate would remain high for the first few hours—something that I knew interfered with quality of sleep and recovery. After experimenting a bit, I now eat my last meal of the day four hours before I go to bed, and this has drastically improved my sleep scores.

Another aspect of my health that I have gained insight into is heart rate variability (HRV). HRV refers to the slight fluctuations or variations in the time between two heartbeats and is considered a good indicator, and even predictor, of heart health. This variability reflects the heart's ability to adapt to different environments and experiences, including periods of stress and relaxation, activity and rest. Higher HRVs indicate better heart and overall health, reflecting the adaptability of the body. The Whoops band is the gold standard for measuring HRV and many athletes swear by how accurately it measures HRV throughout the day and night. When I first started wearing Whoops, my HRV was quite low and it reflected in my readiness score for the next day. Again, I began to experiment with different activities and workouts to see the impact on my heart rate. I figured out that doing more cardio in the day significantly improves HRV. Now, on normal days, my HRV is in the thirties and, on good days, in the early forties, which also reflects in much better Whoop HRV scores.

The advancements in science and cutting-edge technology are truly transforming the world of health. Tracking devices don't just give you measurements of various parameters, but also offer information that could lead to lifestyle changes for better health. In this chapter, we will review the ways in which we can really push the boundaries of health as we know it, leveraging the science and technology now available to become superhuman.

* * *

When we think of health, we think of a sound mind in a sound body, and this, perhaps, is what most of us strive for. We talk about nutrition and exercise, mental health and mindfulness, sleep and freedom from illness. Increasingly, however, with the fascinating advances in the science of human ageing, the scope of health has taken on an entirely new meaning. It's no longer just enough to fight illness and eat right, many serious health scientists and biohackers are now talking about living forever; or, at least, as close to forever as we can get. It may still be too early to believe that these dreams are based on robust science but it is undeniable that our understanding of the ageing process is getting better by the day and some of these biohackers are literally betting their lives on solving the ageing problem. There is no denying that we live in very interesting times and will live to see the mystery of living and dying unfold at an exponentially evolving pace. It is yet to be seen where all this will lead us but I, for one, am in the more optimistic camp and can't wait to see what lies in the future!

One of the most revolutionary ideas in this field is that ageing might not be inevitable. Since growing old has been something we've considered an intrinsic part of life and death for all of human history, this concept has really got the world of science rethinking everything we've ever known about age. In fact, some researchers at the forefront of this area of study have proposed that not only is ageing avoidable, but it is a disease in itself—one that they are now focused on figuring out how to cure.

The field of longevity has come a long way, boasting the work of some very serious biohackers like Dave Asprey and Ben Greenfield as well as renowned scientists like David Sinclair, George Church, Daniel Amen and Aubrey de Grey. They have started to decode the numerous factors that lead to ageing, while exploring and experimenting with potential cures and methods to slow down the process. People in the field have many diverse goals, ranging from slowing down the impact of old age to maintaining full vitality into later years, to drastically extending the human lifespan to anywhere from 125 years to 175 years. This may be hard to imagine today but once we reflect on the fact that the human lifespan has nearly doubled in the last 100 years and that technological breakthroughs continue at an accelerating pace, we are in for a very exciting time ahead. It may be difficult to accurately forecast exactly what to expect, but there is no denying that our age-old notions of age, lifespan and health span are likely to be drastically altered in the coming years.

As we talk about becoming superhumans, chasing longevity and potentially living forever, it's also important to ask why we seek immortality. For most people, until very recently, old age was something to dread. It was synonymous with disease and dysfunction, both physical and mental. Ageing was associated with a gradual loss of memory, cognition, mobility and just about every other bodily function, confining one to a bed, a room, an assisted living home with full time care. Not something to look forward to. And this is why the quest for a longer life now goes hand-in-hand with the quest to live healthier, meaningful lives full of vitality, engagement and zest for life. If we can remain healthy, strong, fit and less susceptible to disease, fractures and other conditions, then perhaps old age doesn't have to be as bad as it's always made out to be. In fact, it might be something to look forward to. Old age could become a time to see through all the projects and dreams of your life; to pursue the hobbies and interests you never had time for; or just to spend with family and grandchildren. For entrepreneurs in Silicon Valley and elsewhere, it could be the opportunity to experience the future of technology, to witness the fruits of one's labours on start-ups, inventions and ideas.

There are, of course, those who say that our planet won't be able to support a population of immortal humans and others who continue to approach old age and death as an inevitable and intrinsic part of the human experience. However, the idea of holding on to one's vitality and quality of life well into old age is a valuable one, that could motivate us to take better care of our bodies and minds as we grow older. As fertility rates decrease, a steady increase in lifespan might be one way to counter the potential population decline. Many developed countries have already reached fertility rates that are well below the rates required to maintain current population levels and many others are expected to follow suit in the coming decades. There is no question that the percentage of people over sixty in the world will continue to increase and we will have to find ways for them to be valued and engaged citizens of the world.

We have always looked at old age as the 'sunset years' with nothing much to do except kick back, reflect and pursue modest goals. But all this is about to change in a major way, with people nurturing the same dreams, ambitions and drive at sixty as they did at twenty, practically looking ahead to another life's worth of learning, exploration and adventure. What can be a better gift than that? Perhaps, British Philosopher Bertrand Russell got it right in his essay, *How to Grow Old*, when he says: 'If you have wide and keen interests and activities in which you can still be effective, you will have no reason to think about the merely statistical fact of the number of years you have already lived, still less of the probable shortness of your future.'[1]

THE UPPER LIMIT OF HUMAN AGE

If indeed ageing is not our unavoidable fate, what is the limit to longevity? Does the human lifespan have limits at all? We currently live almost twice as long as we did back at the turn of the twentieth century, and the current record for longest human life is 122 years and 164 days—a record held by Frenchwoman Jeanne Calment who died in 1997.[2]

A study in 2016 claimed that the human lifespan was fixed at about 115 years, but further research has challenged the idea that there is an upper limit at all when it comes to human age. This was followed by a fascinating study in 2018[3] by demographer Elisabetta Barbi and her colleagues in Italy. The researchers tracked every Italian citizen who had reached the age of 105 between 2009 and 2015, and they found something interesting. It's common knowledge that mortality rates are high in infancy, falling during early childhood and adolescence and then rising again in the thirties until they skyrocket in the seventies and eighties. However, what this study found was that the death rate didn't just keep rising after this. Instead, mortality was found to suddenly flatten at this age. And, in fact, they found that the later people were born, the lower their mortality rate when they reached 105. Therefore, not only was the curve flattening, but the plateau was dipping. This could indicate that we haven't yet reached the maximum human lifespan yet.

The oldest living person in the world as of writing this book in 2022 is a French nun known as Sister Andre who was born in February 1904 and is 118 years old. There are several other supercentenarians, or those who are over 110 years of age, around the world. While science races to discover the secrets of longer life, we can only wait to see the truths that emerge, while following the lives of these incredibly long-lived people from a distance.

First, the Basics

The quest to become superhuman doesn't start with crazy experimental treatments and exotic superfoods. It begins with that most simple and mundane of all things—a healthy lifestyle, followed day after day, year after year and yes, decade after decade. If you are able to do certain things consistently, the power of compounding will start to kick in and you will be surprised by how much small things can add up over a period of time. After looking at all the literature around extreme longevity and performance, the basics always turn out to be the following:

- Sleep: No one enjoys long term good health and vitality without taking sleep very seriously. The body repairs, restores and rejuvenates itself while we are sleeping, so a minimum of seven to eight hours of good quality rest is a must.
- Movement: Adequate movement that takes up the heart rate, combined with resistance and functional training, can slow down the body's eventual decline into the decrepitude of old age.
- Food: If long-term health is your goal, you have no choice but to be very conscious of every morsel of food and drink you consume. A mostly plant-based diet is ideal, with some fasting windows in between—the best anti-ageing antidote known to humankind.
- The Mind: Engaging your mind in worthwhile pursuits that challenge you and are deeply meaningful will keep your mind sharp, leveraging the inherent plasticity of the brain even in older age.
- Being Social: Your life literally depends on other people. Deep, meaningful social connections will go a long way towards cultivating a sense of belongingness, which is a huge factor in living long.

HEALTH HACK #26: Practice Hara Hachi Bu

One of the Japanese secrets to longevity comes from an ancient saying, 'Hara Hachi Bu', which roughly translates to only eating until you're 80 per cent full. So, instead of serving yourself seconds, or eating until you feel stuffed, leave the dining table when you still don't feel completely satiated, and give your digestive system a chance to catch up. It takes about 30–40 minutes for the glucose from food to hit your bloodstream, and about the same time for the brain to signal satiation.

The Obstacles

We have spent enough time covering the modern lifestyle and its implications for our health and vitality. While it is impossible to shun all aspects of modern living and go back to existing like our hunter–gatherer ancestors did, there are a few elements of this lifestyle that pose too many dangers in the long term. If you can bring yourself to reflect on these and give them up, or at least reduce them to the occasional indulgence, it will go a long way in establishing the platform for superhuman capabilities. The following are the biggest dangers to health:

-   Tobacco: Everything that needs to be said about how toxic tobacco can be is now old news, because smoking has almost guaranteed long term negative consequences on health. It is also highly addictive and giving up the habit might require an immense support system and a great deal of willpower.

Everything we discuss in this book becomes redundant if you continue accumulating the damage from a sustained habit of smoking. To live healthier and explore your superhuman potential, you've got to give it up.

- Alcohol: Alcohol has become an integral part of our social lives and no big occasion or gathering seems complete without the customary clink of glasses. But we have come a long way from the pseudo-science that once promoted the health benefits of drinking, and we now know better. Alcohol is bad for long term health and there are no two ways about it. You can certainly have a glass or two occasionally, but anything more regular will have long term consequences.

- Sugar: It took us a long time to unmask the health supervillain that was hiding in plain sight. Sugar is not only a cultural artefact but is also deeply associated with many of our rituals and celebrations. The damage from sugar, however, is all too real and not worth the long-term price that you pay. Shunning sugar in most forms, perhaps allowing yourself only the occasional indulgence, is the best you can do for your body.

Biohacking: The World of DIY Biology

While mainstream science has advanced by leaps and bounds over the last several decades, especially when it comes to health and beyond, some of the most fascinating findings have come from the fringe. This is the world of biohacking—DIY biology that involves stepping beyond traditional science and medicine to experiment with ways of manipulating the mind and the body to optimize performance and health.

While biohackers talk about optimizing, upgrading or taking control of their minds and bodies, the objective for most is, ultimately, deep longevity and the health span to go along with it. Dave Asprey, for example, is on a quest to live to the age of 180! It's not just about living longer, though, but about performing at high levels throughout life, well into old age. To this end, biohackers experiment with everything from diet and nutrition to fitness, mindfulness and supplements to wearable technology and increasingly extreme methods involving ice water immersion, injecting stem cells or transfusing young blood.

Silicon Valley has been at the epicentre of biohacking, taking the idea of self-improvement to an entirely different level. The link between health and productivity at work, now established without a doubt, has brought health into the spotlight for CEOs, start-ups and entrepreneurs. The idea of hacking systems using principles of engineering—something most tech geeks understand—has been adapted to the human body and mind. They have brought an obsession for precision, numbers and quantifying everything to the world of health, transforming the way it is viewed. This might be why wearable tracking devices are so closely related to the world of biohacking—because biohackers rely on measurements of sleep, calories, fitness and pretty much anything else that can be measured.

Biohacking includes everything, from ancient wisdom such as spending time in Vipassana meditation, to common trends such as intermittent fasting. However, some biohackers also use nootropics ('smart drugs'), compounds that are thought to enhance physical or mental performance or insert chips into different parts of their bodies. Many experiment with different supplements, some of them bordering on the bizarre, creating their own concoctions, measuring their exact caffeine intake, finding pills that help them work with better focus or to tide them through periods of jetlag.

Biohackers want to use science and technology to improve the species, but much of what they do hasn't yet been validated by research or approved by medical bodies. This is why, if you're looking forward to trying some of the more exciting hacks, it's best to tread with a little caution. It's important to first understand your body and mind, as well as your goals and requirements, before you leap into the deep end. It is also equally important to get the basics right first. If your fundamentals are not in the right place, the extreme measures of biohacking will do you no good and may even be harmful. It's a thrilling world, however, and with some of the popular biohackers' books, podcasts and blogs, you can find a guide to lead you through it.

THERAPIES FOR SUPERHUMANS

Many of the less invasive techniques to boost performance, access longevity and hack the health of the body that are practised by biohackers are becoming available to lay people, and are now being offered by centres in India.

One treatment for ageing that has grown popular is IV infusion therapy, which involves the direct delivery of essential vitamins and nutrients into the bloodstream. The levels of these substances in the blood go up to levels that are higher than normal, leading to a therapeutic effect including reversing deficiencies that could cause disorders. The infusion can be customized to an individual's needs, boosting energy, stimulating the immune system, improving sleep and helping to manage stress.

Hyperbaric Oxygen Therapy (HBOT) is a treatment used to enhance the body's natural healing processes. This therapy is administered in a chamber with almost pure oxygen where air pressure is increased to allow the lungs to breathe in this concentrated oxygen. As a result, the amount of oxygen carried by the blood increases, while plasma, lymph and other fluids also carry oxygen to damaged tissues or regions of the body where circulation is blocked. HBOT has effects at the cellular level, promoting healing and boosting cellular pathways associated with health and longevity.

Restricted Environment Stimulation Therapy (REST) works on the same principle as sensory deprivation, using flotation tanks filled with water and Epsom salts. Floating in this device blocks out 90 per cent of the environmental stimulation that would affect the body, suppressing the fight-or-flight stress response of the sympathetic nervous system and boosting the relaxation response of the parasympathetic nervous system. REST helps hack into the elusive 'theta' state, one that is highly meditative and creative, boosting neurological connections.

One of the defining characteristics of old age is the loss of muscle tissue and strength, which, in turn, causes frailty and increases the risk for a range of illnesses and injuries. This is why the EMSculpt, a device using focused electromagnetic energy to trigger supramaximal muscle contractions—contractions greater than those which can be achieved through voluntary action—might work as a therapy for longevity. While it is currently promoted as a weight loss and body contouring treatment for toned and firm muscles, it has great potential to prevent diabetes, boost immunity, strengthen the bones and address many symptoms of ageing.

Our blood contains platelets, red and white blood cells, as well as plasma, some of which contains high concentrations of platelets. In a new form of therapy, a patient's blood is drawn and put through a centrifuge, after which this 'platelet-rich plasma' or PRP is reintroduced via an injection. Platelets are high in growth factors, nutrients and proteins that can reduce pain and inflammation. PRP therapy is most effective for acute conditions like injuries and osteoarthritis, while also regenerating the tissues of the face and the skin.

These are just a few of the more exciting treatments and therapies that are now more easily available to us, and there are plenty more. We live in a time of constant new research and the development of cutting-edge technologies that are beginning to transform how we view health. As always, it is best to not only do your own research but also to check with your doctor before trying anything new, especially if you suffer from any condition.

LEARNING LIKE A MAESTRO

Science and technology have truly raised the bar and changed the game for performance training, just as they have in so many other fields of health. Neuropriming is based on the understanding that the brain can and should be harnessed to unlock and optimize performance potential. Given the incredibly profound connection between the brain and the body, it seems obvious that the brain must be addressed when trying to achieve peak potential. While practices like meditation are a great way of tapping into focus, handling stress or improving cognition, neuropriming goes a step further, by stimulating parts of the brain associated with movement using an electric current. The scientific term for this is transcranial direct current stimulation.

The most well-known neuropriming device is the Halo Sport. It leverages the neuroplasticity of the brain to tap into the parts of it involved in learning movement and motor skills. The device resembles a headset, and delivers neurostimulation to the brain, in order to boost the neural pathways in the motor cortex. This results in accelerated learning, better muscle memory and more efficient practice sessions. High performers and elite athletes have reported that using a Halo Sport just before a session gets them straight into the zone—a feeling they would otherwise experience twenty or thirty minutes into a training session.

Essentially, what the Halo device and other similar technologies do, is boost the neuroplasticity of the brain. Each time we learn a new motor skill, our brain develops the neural pathways for that skill, whether it's throwing a ball in a certain way, or strumming chords on a guitar in a particular pattern. Neuropriming stimulates the brain to increase the firing of the neurons in a pathway so that the development of that pathway speeds up, making the practice that follows more efficient. Neuropriming takes the brain into a heightened state of neuroplasticity, known as hyper plasticity.

Several peer-reviewed published papers have found that neuropriming using the Halo Sport device can indeed be effective, with results varying from a 15 per cent improvement in running endurance, to a 60 per cent acceleration of fine motor skills learning and significantly enhanced performance in sprint cyclists. Neuropriming is in no way a replacement for or alternative to serious practice and training. It can only create a brain that is more open to learning and offer the opportunity for better, quicker and more accurate learning, as well as more efficient practice.

Another recent discovery in the science of learning is the effect of increased cortisol, or the stress response, on learning. It comes from the simple observation that out in the wild, if we have a scary experience, our brain remembers every small detail so that if we ever encounter that situation again, we will be well prepared. This phenomenon can be hacked to accelerate learning by activating your peripheral nervous system (PNS) through activities like exercise, cold exposure and heat exposure. Some biohackers might engage in a quick sprint or a set of burpees before they set out to learn something and then harness that state of arousal to sharpen their focus and retention. Another great technique to boost retention is to take a nap after a few hours of intense study to boost long term memory formation. You can take it to the next level by designing a study protocol that involves vigorous exercise followed by a long learning session, and then ensuring you get a good night's sleep before recalling the concepts again, first thing in the morning. You will be surprised by how this protocol can dramatically accelerate long term retention and the wiring of new neural circuits.

NOOTROPICS

For most lay people, until recently, ageing was discussed and addressed in terms of its physical aspects—face creams to target wrinkles, hair dyes to hide sneaky greys and other cosmetic quick fixes to make us look younger. The latest research, however, has dived far deeper into the study of ageing—how to slow it down and even reverse it—than ever before. Beyond physical appearance and even physiological processes, a big symptom of ageing as we now know it is cognitive decline. This is where a new class of 'smart drugs' or 'cognitive enhancers' known as nootropics comes in. The word has Greek roots, literally meaning 'to bend or shape the mind'.

While we might associate forgetfulness and confusion with people in their eighties and nineties, the truth is that the slowing down in brain function starts much earlier. There is some evidence to show that the gradual deterioration in our intellectual abilities might begin as early as in our twenties, while the volume of the brain starts to decrease in our forties. Nootropics promise to slow down or perhaps even reverse this decline by boosting higher level brain function including memory, motivation, decision-making, concentration and even creativity. These drugs work by crossing the blood–brain barrier, providing the brain with essential nutrients, boosting blood circulation and blood flow to the brain, increasing energy levels, and reducing inflammation. Some nootropics take the form of naturally occurring substances, while other supplements and pills—most available over the counter—are synthesized in a lab.

While research into nootropics is still in its early stages, some substances and ingredients have been proven to have brain boosting properties. Known as the 'king herb' from Chinese medicine, ginseng contains an active compound that affects the central nervous system, improving mental performance and aspects of memory.[4] Brahmi, also known as Bacopa monnieri, is a nootropic that Ayurveda swears by. This compound stimulates and enhances the memory and intellect by combining the chemical constituents of bacosides A and B. They facilitate learning, speeding up mental processing and improving retention. I like brahmi for its multifaceted roles in protecting the liver from damage and acting as an anticancer, antistress and anti-addiction agent, in addition to its cognitive enhancing abilities. Another much loved herb of Ayurvedic medicine is ashwagandha, also known as Withania somnifera, which has been used as a nerve tonic for its effects on the central nervous system as well as its antistress and anti-ageing properties.

The extract of the Ginkgo biloba tree that grows in China has been studied for its ability to increase blood flow to the brain and improve memory, both in healthy patients as well as in those with dementia.

Rhodiola rosea is another well-known nootropic, also known as the golden or arctic root, which grows in the mountains of

Europe and Asia, and has been used in traditional medicine for hundreds of years. This plant has powerful properties that make it a cognitive enhancer, boosting memory and learning, while protecting the nervous system from degradation and stabilizing emotions. All these offer various forms of protection against the ageing of the brain, making them powerful ingredients in our quest for becoming superhuman.

In addition to the naturally occurring ingredients, we've discussed above, there are drugs like modafinil, originally prescribed for narcolepsy and sleep disorders, but now used by many as a cognitive enhancer—its benefits are believed to include improved pattern recognition and executive planning. Supplementing with certain non-essential amino acids like L-theanine, L-tyrosine, L-taurine and Acetyl-L- carnitine also work as cognitive enhancers, by boosting cellular energy production and, in turn, improving levels of neurotransmitters like dopamine and noradrenaline.

Nootropic stacks or a combination of nootropics always yield better results than those taken in isolation. These smart drugs address everything from brain fog and difficulty in concentration or memory to improving mental strength to be at the top of your game as an athlete. It's a good idea to speak to a doctor or nutritionist to help figure out the dose and type of nootropics best for you based on your age, medical conditions, and goals.

While nootropics are a fascinating area of research, it's good to remember that their perks for the brain are cumulative, which means you need to take them consistently over fairly long periods of time to experience their effects. Many people prefer to boost their brain health the old school way, by increasing intake of fish, berries, brightly coloured and pigmented fruits and vegetables, or by drinking herb concoctions as daily elixirs. Don't forget that there really are no magic pills when it comes to health, and even the most powerful nootropic cannot be used as an alternative to a healthy lifestyle that includes regular exercise, sufficient restful sleep and a diet of real, plant-based foods.

HEALTH HACK #27: Ashwagandha

Ashwagandha is an Ayurvedic herb that has been used for thousands of years for its adaptogenic properties—helping the body resist stress. It has been prescribed as a tonic for wide-ranging benefits, from boosting energy, strength and vitality, to treating inflammation, depression, digestive problems and more.

BUILDING SUPERPOWERS

In the last two decades, one of the most successful movie franchises has been *The Avengers* series, which brings together a whole cast of superheroes with amazing powers to fight exotic villains and save the world, time and time again. Some of these superheroes have mutations that give them incredible powers and the stories are lapped up by billions around the world. Perhaps they stoke some of our own fantasies about having superpowers, and we vicariously enjoy the thrill of flying through space, swinging from bridges and seamlessly travelling across many realms. In short, we are utterly fascinated by the idea of superpowers, and it is no wonder that Superman and Wonder Woman are some of the most loved comic book and film characters.

The world of superpowers doesn't end with just these fictional characters, however. We see incredible feats of human endurance in sport, especially extreme sports. When Eliud Kipchoge attempted to break the two-hour barrier for a full marathon, the whole world was cheering him on, as it signified the transcendence of what we had always considered an insurmountable boundary of human performance. When he successfully broke the record, we all collectively celebrated another step forward for all of humanity. And then, there is Wim Hof, who climbs snowy peaks wearing nothing but shorts—making it look like a walk in the park. The Netflix documentary, *14 Peaks,* brought to the spotlight the Nepali mountaineer Nims Purja who summited the world's fourteen highest peaks in just seven months—when the previous record for this endeavour was eight years! Extreme athletes in sports such as solo climbing, free diving and surfing pull off stunts that seem to defy the laws of physics and the limits of what the human body can do.

These superpowers are not only limited to feats of physical endurance. Indian yogis have garnered a great deal of attention in the last few decades for their almost magical ability to slow down their heart rates, increase their body temperature at will and get their brains into trance-like states on demand. These yogis have been studied by neuroscience labs around the world, and the profound potential of deep meditation and breathing techniques to achieve altered states of consciousness is just beginning to be understood.

The story of Yongey Mingyur Rinpoche, a Tibetan Buddhist teacher and an expert meditator, illustrates the ways in which the human mind can voluntarily access deep meditative states, bringing about profound changes in the brain. With over 60,000 hours of meditation, Mingyur has more lifetime hours of practice than most other people, and this is what made the scientists at the University of Wisconsin-Madison want to look deep inside his brain. During the first EEG scan conducted in 2002, researchers were shocked to see the sudden and dramatic burst of electrical activity in Mingyur's brain every time he was instructed to engage in compassion. These spikes decreased but did not vanish even during periods of mental rest. This was the first time such brain activity during meditation was observed in a lab setting. When Mingyur's brain was scanned in an fMRI, the results were even more stunning—during periods of compassion meditation, his brain circuitry for empathy rose to 700–800 per cent more than it had been when his mind was at rest.

Mingyur's brain was scanned one more time in 2010, before he announced that he was going on a retreat again—a tradition of Tibetan monks where they become wandering yogis, spending over three years in meditation. For the next four years he all but disappeared, spending the colder months in the plains of India, while retreating to Himalayan caves when the weather grew warmer. After this extended period of solitude, Mingyur next returned to the lab in 2016. With the three MRI scans the researchers now had, they were able to look at age-related declines in grey matter density, using various landmarks to estimate the age of the brain. Using this technique, scientists are able to compare a person's chronological age with the age of their brain. And Mingyur, at the age of forty-one, had the brain of a thirty-three-year-old. While people's brains age at different rates, this was a significant finding. Further studies on Mingyur and other yogis found that they all had unusual baseline brain waves, in which gamma waves were sustained for minutes at a time rather than the split seconds experienced by non-meditators and beginners. In addition, the yogis and monks had a much lower response to the anticipation of pain, experiencing the actual pain momentarily and then recovering from it very quickly. This means they are able to fully experience and respond to challenging situations, without the interference of worry, anxiety or other emotional reactions.

Some of these superpowers stem from the ability of practitioners—both extreme athletes and yogis—to be able to transcend the division of the mind between conscious thought and subconscious processes. This is a concept that Scott Carney delves into in his book, *The Wedge*.[5] This term refers to the fleeting moment or space between what happens to the body and how we choose to react to it. For example, imagine getting a vaccine in your thigh. Instinctively, you're likely to flinch, even before the shot, knowing that you're going to feel the poke. When the needle pierces your flesh, an electric signal is triggered, which takes a few microseconds to travel to the brain. The brain interprets the signal as a potentially harmful event, triggering a pain response that might include a scream, jerking away, or even tears. But if you pause and think about it, it is merely an electric signal. What if you could train your mind to ignore that signal? That's exactly what world class endurance athletes do, as do experienced meditators. They can create the distance or the 'Wedge' between a stimulus travelling to the brain and choosing the response. If you become very good at it—and it takes a lot of practice to get there—you can start to demonstrate superhuman traits that you wouldn't have thought possible.

Our modern lives have made us creatures of comfort. If we're too hot we can turn on the air-conditioning, if we're even the slightest bit hungry we can order a snack and, if we want to, we can spend all day in various luxuriously cushioned pieces of furniture, so that discomfort is a feeling we're barely acquainted with. And yet, to push through the barriers of human potential, to achieve new heights of physical and mental performance and to become superhuman, we must step much further out of our comfort zones than we are used to. It is by tapping into the Wedge, this little gap, and taking control of the autonomous or conditioned response, that humans have achieved incredible feats of endurance. With the Wedge, we can build resilience and endurance, making better decisions instead of running away from the first signs of pain. By exposing ourselves to extreme temperatures and other less-than-comfortable environments and experiences, we're learning to take control of our responses to these situations, both physically and psychologically. From running hundreds of miles to immersing themselves into ice cold water for minutes, to holding their breath for over ten minutes—seemingly ordinary humans are able to perform these herculean feats by reaching into this space in the mind that governs the response to external stimuli.

The immense power of controlled stress to boost growth has been known since ancient times. The adage 'no pain no gain', Nietzsche's proclamation that, 'What doesn't kill you makes you stronger', and the writings of ancient stoics who extolled the virtues of obstacles being the greatest source of growth, all stem from this insight. Author Ryan Holiday expounds on this theme in his book *The Obstacle is the Way*, whose core idea is that we need obstacles, major life challenges and extreme situations, to push beyond our limits, find new capabilities that we never realized we had or could develop and come away stronger and wiser from the experience. Biohackers are now taking the same idea into the modern age by harnessing various artificial stressors from heat and cold to endurance sports to multi-day fasting, all to trigger very powerful body responses, thus hacking biology to perform at extraordinarily high levels that go beyond what is considered normal or is comfortable.

Several meditation and mindfulness techniques have been found to alter the functioning of our brains, offering us another way into the Wedge or a way to hack our psychological response to challenging situations. For example, Jon Kabat-Zin, who created the Mindfulness-Based Stress Reduction Programme (MBSR), found that meditation techniques that increased self-awareness could help separate the emotional experience of pain from the cognitive. The brains of experienced meditators showed less reactivity to stress, particularly in the amygdala, the part of the brain which activates the fight-or-flight response. This means that meditation techniques could help make us more resilient to stress, an important superpower for our arsenal.

Many of the superpowers we strive for rest on the powerful connection between our minds and bodies. Tales from the Himalayas tell of mysterious Tibetan Buddhist monks who have been practicing Tummo or 'inner fire' meditation for thousands of years. Legends claim that these seasoned meditators could melt circles in the snow around them from the immense body heat that they could generate on demand, while others could survive the freezing temperatures in nothing but thin, single layers of clothing. The Tummo techniques have been adapted and are now used by high performers, including professional surfers and MMA fighters, to get themselves into the zone, as well as by people suffering from chronic pain and stress. In fact, Wim Hof's technique borrows from Tummo, releasing neurochemicals and hormones that downregulate inflammation while boosting immune cell production.

The foundation for becoming 'superhuman' boils down to a healthy lifestyle. The superpowers you might be striving for are nothing but the sum of the small daily habits that you must build, gradually achieving a transformation, both within and without.

HARNESSING THE MAGIC OF STEM CELLS

What could possibly be common between a neuron in the brain and a white blood cell that fights infections? A muscle fibre cell looks so different from a retinal cell which can sense light and convert it into an electric signal to be interpreted as an image by the brain. We not only have this amazing complexity and variety among our cells, but also retain the ability to regenerate almost all our cells throughout our adult lives. It is this ability to grow new cells that allows our broken bones to heal, new learning to happen via new neuronal circuits, blood to get replenished after we donate blood or new muscle cells to grow in response to weight training. How do all these new cells grow?

The cells responsible for this seemingly miraculous ability are known as stem cells, which have the potential to develop into any specialized cell with the right trigger. There are two types of stem cells: embryonic and adult. As the name suggests, embryonic stem cells are responsible for the development of a foetus into a baby. An embryonic stem cell is pluripotent, meaning that it can develop into any cell of the adult human body. The complexity involved in this specialization is mind-boggling and it will take a while before we understand every step and signal in complete detail. Until then, and luckily for you and me, this process works flawlessly! Adult stem cells are found in almost all parts of the body and spring into action every time a tissue needs to be repaired or a damaged cell needs to be replaced.

Not long ago, scientists thought stem cells only existed at the embryonic stage, and with their ability to morph into any kind of cell, the possibilities for organ regeneration and novel cures for several diseases opened. This started a gold rush in stem cell research alongside a quest to find pristine stem cells as raw material. One source of embryonic stem cells turned out to be fertilization clinics, where people would freeze early-stage embryos, some of which didn't end up being used in pregnancies. The use of stem cells derived from these embryos caused a political storm in the

USA, eventually leading to a ban on embryonic stem cell research, and potentially setting back the pace of progress by a decade. Fortunately, it became possible to extract adult stem cells from fat cells and the spinal cord, which put research back on track. Since then, it has gone ahead full steam and many novel stem cell therapies are already hitting the trial stage.

As an expecting parent you might have seen brochures about storing a newborn's placenta, in order to save the body's embryonic stem cells for use in cures that might be developed. But now, with much improved techniques available to harvest adult stem cells, it is not as important.

There are already ways of banking your stem cells while you're still young and vigorous, so that you have access to that young and vigorous version of yourself even as you grow older. This is still a fairly expensive practice, but is likely to become more affordable as medical technology develops. If you suffer from a major injury, get cancer, diabetes or any other disease that could be life threatening, being able to access your stem cells could make a huge difference to your recovery. According to biohacker Dave Asprey, there are a few hacks to boost stem cell activity in your body. These include boron supplements, doing occasional twenty-four-hour fasts or other forms of calorie restriction, restricting sugar intake, lifting weights and taking turmeric supplements. In addition, he recommends resveratrol supplements, vitamins D3 and C, doing tai chi exercises and spending more time in nature.

Stem cells might be the single most important cell in human life, for their ability to literally build the rest of the body. The study of stem cells and their incredible capacity is now one of the most exciting areas of health research, with numerous possibilities for therapies and treatments. Stem cell therapies are starting to get a lot of attention due to their immense potential for regenerative medicine, accelerating healing, regenerating tissues and, perhaps someday, leading to complete organ transplants with no chance of rejection, as it would be exactly your own DNA.

The application of stem cell therapy is vast and has the potential to transform medicine, from recovery and healing to anti-ageing. Thanks to the ability of stem cells to become neurons, muscle cells and other kinds of tissue, they play a significant role in recovery and the regeneration of injured, dysfunctional or ageing tissues. Stem cells might also play an important role in drug testing. Considering that the decline in number and function of stem cells is one of the hallmarks of ageing, stem cell therapy can be used to slow down or pause this process. The reason stem cells might act as a biological clock is because, as we age, we increasingly draw on our reserve of stem cells, especially from the bone marrow, for repair and recovery—this is even more true for those who suffer chronic illness or who have undergone intensive training as athletes.

Back to the Future

The future of healthcare is already here, and it is absolutely thrilling to be able to witness it. Here is just a glimpse of some of the therapies, procedures and ideas that are being researched and tested, and might soon be available to us:

Restorative & Preventive Therapy

Progenitor stem cells are descendants of embryonic stem cells and are able to differentiate into cells that replenish blood and marrow cells, repair the central nervous system, keep skin and hair healthy, as well as become cells of the muscles, bones, ligaments and tendons. The Wnt signalling pathways of the body—a particular group of chemical reactions, molecules and proteins that allow cell-to-cell communication—have been found to influence embryonic development as well as carcinogenesis or the formation of cancers, and these pathways seem to go haywire with age. Biosplice is an organization that hacks these two biological mechanisms—creating medicines and devices that target stem cells using the Wnt pathways. Their molecules dial up certain cells to restore and rejuvenate tissues, while dialling down others to treat tumours. Early tests have been promising, and they are working on devices, medicines and molecules to address osteoarthritis, solid and liquid tumours, Alzheimer's, tendinitis, degenerative disc disease, chronic lung scarring and male pattern baldness.

CANCER TREATMENT

Chimeric Antigen Response T-cell (CAR-T) therapy combines immunotherapy and gene therapy and might be at the pinnacle of personalized medicine. Cancer cells often go under the radar of our immune system's T-cells, especially as we age. In a laboratory, a patient's own T-cells are genetically engineered with a special receptor, called the chimeric antigen response, to bind to proteins on certain cancer cells, identifying and then attacking them. These CAR T-cells then persist in the patient's body after the therapy. Carl June, the American immunologist who developed this 'living drug' believes that soon, CAR T-cell therapy and similar immunotherapies will be the frontline of cancer treatment, rather than chemotherapy.

Treating Parkinson's Disease

Unfortunately, the current frontline treatment for Parkinson's Disease is not always effective for all patients, and when it is, the side effects are still unpleasant. A new technology known as focused ultrasound, however, might transform the lives of people living with Parkinson's. Insightec, a medical device company, has developed this technology, which consists of high energy sound waves, precision guided by MRIs. In tests, it has been found to alleviate symptoms without the need for incisions or anaesthesia with resulting risks for infection. It not only reduces tremors, but also restores critical function.

Precision Medicine

Artificial intelligence is already revolutionizing medicine, and what was once the stuff of science fiction, like tiny robot doctors, is now turning to reality. Bionaut Labs has developed remote-controlled 'microbots', each smaller than a single grain of rice, which can be inserted into the body to deliver precision drugs. This has the potential to transform our approach to treatments for diseases like cancer, which, though localized, are targeted with things like chemotherapy that affect the entire body. The accuracy of Bionaut's tiny robots is equivalent to that of surgeons, redefining the very meaning of precision medicine.

Regenerative Medicine

Exosomes are extracellular vesicles which can be likened to tiny bubbles that stem cells release. These carry genetic information and proteins through the body, forming a communication pathway between cells. Exosomes are extracted from human mesenchymal stem cells that have the power to differentiate into different cell types, and then administered through IV or injection. Exosomes improve cellular communication, reduce inflammation and boost regeneration of damaged cells. The healing powers of exosomes can be harnessed for the treatment of chronic inflammation and pain, including conditions like osteoarthritis and musculoskeletal injuries. Their regenerative powers and positive effects on the immune system mean that they also play a role in anti-ageing.

ADVANCED DIAGNOSTICS

Alongside medical therapies and technologies, diagnostics have also advanced by leaps and bounds, allowing us to take our health into our hands like never before. Cleerly is a new coronary CT angiography guided by artificial intelligence to differentiate between safe and dangerous plaque found in a heart scan—since calcified cholesterol plaques are stable and don't pose a risk, while soft plaques are more likely to rupture. Not only can this technology prevent heart attacks, it can also prevent unnecessary invasive heart procedures. Through a simple blood test, the GRAIL test can detect more than fifty types of cancer. Combined with a full body MRI, it can detect a complete spectrum of early-stage cancers, which have an 89 per cent chance of survival, compared to 21 per cent in late stages. AI technology can now analyse brain tissue to determine early signs of Alzheimer's and Parkinson's, gauging whether parts of the brain have increased or decreased in size. When it comes to blood tests, there are now labs measuring over fifty different markers, including vitamin and nutrient levels, insulin, cholesterol, inflammation, hormones and heavy metals, all of which have an impact on health and longevity. To complete this list, there are also bone density tests, DNA and microbiome analyses, skin analyses and AI facial imaging to determine skin health and age.

These are just the tip of the iceberg that is the future of healthcare, and I hope this excites you enough to follow the research coming from the cutting edge.

CENTRES FOR EXTREME HEALTH

A lot of what we have covered in this chapter might sound like something out of a science fiction film, but the truth is that the future of science is here now. While research goes on, biohackers are taking their health into their own hands and bringing their successful experiments to the public—through books, podcasts and blogs, of course, but now, also through real life clinics.

The data that biohackers gather through constant trial and error, pushing the boundaries of the unknown and exploring the possibilities for health, could eventually be used to create apps, so that all of us can become biohackers in our own ways, from home. Following are some of the advanced health centres around the world, with access to the latest and greatest in human longevity, performance treatments and therapies.

1. Upgrade Labs

In the next generation of biohacking, it's likely that lay people will have access to some of the most cutting-edge technology available in a setting not unlike a gym. In fact, Dave Asprey, one of the most well recognized names in the field, has already launched his Upgrade Labs, touted as the world's first biohacking facility. The Lab looks at biomarkers across the brain, body and the function of systems, in order to address health on a cellular level and, in turn, improve longevity. Asprey himself claims to have spent over a million dollars on experimenting with technology, supplements and various kinds of treatments, and his facility is a way of making some of these more accessible to people pursuing performance in the long term.

The Upgrade Lab offers services across recovery, performance and cognitive improvements, addressing everything from immunity, inflammation and sleep, to toxins, longevity and peak performance. For recovery, clients can pick cryotherapy, an infrared sauna, an atmospheric cell trainer and something called the 'big squeeze', among others. To boost performance, the options include cold HIIT and a device known as the 'cheat machine', while a virtual flotation tank offers clarity of thought and deep meditation. At the moment, Asprey's Upgrade Lab is expensive, with two branches in Santa Monica and the Beverly Hills in California, but it seems as though the future holds a lot more in store for us.

2. Next Health

Another brand making the latest health technology more accessible is Next Health, with centres for health optimization and longevity. Here, you can undergo a battery of tests to determine everything from gut health and food sensitivities to micronutrient levels and genetic health. Based on your biomarkers, you could have a wellness plan created for you to boost your vitality and your longevity. The services included IV drips and vitamin shots that promise to boost energy, alleviate stress and even cure hangovers! In addition, clients can try out cryotherapy or infrared light therapy, as well as ozone therapy and hormone optimization. There are also offerings for aesthetic services such as skin tightening and 'wrinkle relaxers'.

Next Health positions itself as a place that allows clients to take their health into their own hands, rather than wait for something to go wrong before seeking medical intervention. And while the centres are run by medical professionals, they are marketed as 'vibrant' spaces for wellness and social connection.

3. Health Nucleus by Human Longevity Inc

Health Nucleus has created a precision health care programme that harnesses the power of health data to help you optimize your health. Through their 100+ programme, Health Nucleus offers annual assessments that analyse your genomics, blood biomarkers and body imaging. With this enormous quantity of highly precise data, physicians and experts are able to determine the right nutrition, fitness and lifestyle programmes for every client. The entire programme is based on the premise that data, combined with the latest technology, can help detect and prevent disease, thus improving health as well as longevity.

The in-depth diagnostics offered by Health Nucleus includes MRIs, genome sequencing, a whole battery of tests to determine cardiac health, balance tracking, insulin sensitivity testing and body composition analysis, among several others.

4. Medical Spas

Medical spas have become sought after wellness destinations that combine traditional spa methods with medical facilities or expertise, for holistic health and beauty. Europe is home to many luxurious resort spas that offer a range of therapies, from detox routines to massages and saunas. Many of these places come equipped with excellent facilities such as swimming pools, running tracks, meditation rooms and kitchens that prepare nutritious food tailored to clients' needs. The spas have in-house medical professionals, who customize and administer various therapies and track your progress.

HEALTH HACK #28: Biosensor Ink Tattoos

Having a tattoo has never been quite as cool as it is with biosensor ink that changes colour in response to levels of glucose, albumin and pH levels. Still in testing stages, this ink could have wide application in monitoring patients with diabetes or kidney disease.

CHASING IMMORTALITY

For as long as there has been storytelling—which is perhaps as long as our species has existed—there have been legends and myths about the search for eternal life. From Gilgamesh's epic quest in the great Mesopotamian legend, to Tithonus who was granted eternal life but wasted away because his beloved, Eos, did not think to ask for eternal youth, to the search for the Holy Grail by the Knights of the Round Table, immortality was the metaphorical treasure every adventurer and hero sought. Sometimes they achieved it but at a terrible cost, and sometimes they died trying.

The modern pursuit for longevity might not seem very different, and yet it is. While the heroes of legend sought a secret for eternal life in the world around them—an object, a fountain of youth, a secret source in the wilderness—our current day heroes search within. By transforming the way our minds and bodies work, by carefully contemplating everything we consume, how we move, how we sleep, how we recover and tracking every element of our that health that we can, we are taking steps towards living longer lives. The modern-day seeker of immortality has a more detailed map than those of stories and legends.

HEALTH HACK #29: CRISPR

CRISPR is a technology that is used for genome editing—rewriting DNA sequences and modifying the function of genes. The tool can be used to correct genetic defects, as well as in cancer immunotherapy and tissue regeneration. In addition, it might have applications in disease resistance.

IMMORTAL CELLS

The incredible power of our cells is immortalized in the amazing story of Henrietta Lacks, an African-American woman who died of cervical cancer in the 1950s. Cancer is a disease of mutation in which, due to genetic changes, the cells keep dividing uncontrollably. One of the doctors treating Henerietta had removed some of her cancerous cells, and later observed that these cells continued to divide and double every twenty-four hours in the cellular medium in the lab. This division seemed to have no limit, unlike normal cells of the human body, including the most cancerous ones, which eventually stop dividing.

A scientist named George Gey at the same hospital came across these cells and recognized their immense potential in research. He started creating large quantities of the cells and shipping them to various research centres around the world. This cell line has come to be called HeLa, after the first two letters of her first and last names. The cells continue to live and divide even sixty years after Henrietta's death and play an immensely significant role in research around the world. This is just one example of the unknown properties that lie dormant within our genetic code, which a chance mutation might spring to life. As we understand the workings of stem cells and our own genetic code more, we can harness this knowledge for novel treatments and lifestyle changes to stay youthful and vibrant through our adult lives.

Some of the best minds in the world are working on unravelling the mystery of ageing, and as they pursue the ambitious goal of curing ageing, they are piling up one impressive breakthrough after another. The founders of Google have funded a company called Calico Labs, whose explicit purpose is to cure ageing. The similarly heavily funded Human Longevity Institute has undertaken advanced genomic research to find potential solutions to radically alter what we think of as a healthy lifespan. We have only seen the teaser so far, but studies in which the lifespans of lab animals have been extended by 50 per cent might hold the key to a future for humans that we can barely fathom today. In Ray Kurzweil's highly influential book *Fantastic Voyage*, in which he predicted that over a few decades, medical technology would advance so far that every year of living would coincide with an average of a one year increase in lifespan.

We may not be able to predict when and how much the human lifespan will increase but it is a safe bet to say that many of us alive today can expect to live to the age of 100 to 125 years and perhaps even longer (that is, if you don't manage to kill yourself with a lifestyle disease before). These possibilities have immense implications for how you live your life and what choices you make. Many of the old models of ageing, retirement and gracefully walking into the sunset may not apply, and we may have to rethink our lives on a very different timescale. Whether living very long is on your wish list or not, we need to be aware of the possibilities that loom on the horizon and the best way to be ready for and benefit from these breakthroughs is to adapt the most commonsensical approach to a healthy lifestyle.

In Summary

Keep in Mind

1. As humans live longer lives, it is becoming apparent that we do not really know the upper limit of human age.
2. The three biggest obstacles to a better life and health span are tobacco, alcohol and sugar.
3. Currently on the fringe, many biohackers treat their bodies and minds like machines, using data and technology to optimize them for longer life and better health.
4. From IV infusion therapies and sensory deprivation to plasma treatments, many treatments for health and longevity are now easily available in India.
5. By supercharging our brains to boost learning using cutting-edge technology, we can achieve peak potential, not just of our minds but our bodies too.
6. Nootropics are substances and ingredients that have brain-boosting properties, and are valuable for their role in slowing down or reversing cognitive decline with age.
7. As we pursue the next level of health and chase immortality, many of the superpowers we need come from the powerful connection between brain and body.
8. Stem cells have enormous potential in the future of health, giving us access to younger versions of ourselves even as we age.
9. Some of the most futuristics sounding therapies might soon be at the frontline of medical treatment—from microbots to genetically engineered immune cells that can recognize and destroy cancer cells.

10. As longevity becomes a solution many of us seek, there are clinics and centres springing up that offer cutting-edge therapies to boost health and help us live longer.
11. Whether you believe it or not, many people alive today are likely to live to anywhere between 100 and 125.

Take Action

1. In order to become 'superhuman', living a longer and healthier life, you have to get the basics right: better sleep, regular movement, good quality nutrition, an engaged mind and deep social connections.
2. There is really no choice but to give up smoking if you want good health, while alcohol and sugar will have to become rare indulgences.
3. Invest in a good health tracking device if you're keen to tune into your body's metrics and try different ways of influencing them.
4. Speak to your nutritionist or doctor if you would like to try a nootropic or smart drug to boost your brain and protect against cognitive decline.
5. If you'd like to have a super clear dashboard for your health, look up some of the cutting-edge health clinics that you could visit to do a whole battery of tests.
6. Keep up to date by following some of the best biohackers in the world—through their blogs, podcasts, and books.

CONCLUSION

It is said that 'how we spend our days is, of course, how we spend our lives'. When it comes to the journey of health, nothing could be more apt. The story of health unfolds one day at a time and what you do every day slowly but surely adds up. If you suffer from a lifestyle disease, it may not be because you ate one too many cakes last year, but because of a slow accumulation of wear and tear that affected your fat metabolism and insulin regulation when you were in your twenties and thirties. If you start to notice a decline in your mental faculties in your sixties, it is probably because of how little you engaged your brain to pursue good brain health.

What you do everyday matters and the only way to pursue a good lifestyle is by paying attention to how every normal day unfolds. Now, that doesn't mean that every single day counts so much that even an occasional day of bingeing signals that you have completely fallen off the wagon. In fact, the reverse is true. What matters is what you do on 80–90 per cent of your days because those days play a crucial role in wiring your biological and neurological machinery. And if you get these 80–90 per cent of days right, you almost earn the licence to do whatever you want for the remaining day of the week. No one has ever said that the pursuit of good health means that you have to be an absolute disciplinarian and deprive yourself of all the pleasures of life. If you are able to have five or six good or healthy days in a week, you can let your hair down and indulge in whatever gives you joy on the seventh day without causing long term damage.

Sometimes people use the excuse, 'you live only once', to do whatever they want, however they want. They may be able to get by on a few hours of sleep every night and proclaim, 'I will sleep when I am dead.' Just because we have a short lifespan, doesn't mean that you need to cut it down further by poor lifestyle choices! It is no fun to go through the last few decades of life bedridden, saddled with medical bills and having to eat every meal without salt or sugar. The choice of living it up in your twenties and thirties unfortunately comes at the cost of being dependent on others and spending all your savings on medical bills in old age.

The good news is that it doesn't need to be an either–or choice. Healthy habits can make life extraordinarily enjoyable, allowing you to accomplish your life's work. Among modern-day heroes are film stars like Tom Cruise and Akshay Kumar, who are pushing sixty, and Meryl Streep, who is in her seventies, and they're all still going strong. Amitabh Bachchan is still among the top actors in Bollywood as he enters his eighties, and I think we can count on him holding that position for another decade at least! In cricket, we have athletes like James Anderson, one of the top test bowlers in the world in his forties, while those many years his junior cannot think beyond T20s. Good health provides a strong foundation to achieve anything you want to—with more energy and confidence, and with the resilience to bounce back from occasional setbacks or indulgences. What is even better, is that you can continue to enjoy a life of energy and action well into your older years and enjoy the wisdom of old age as much as you enjoyed the wilder years of your youth!

When it comes to the pursuit of good health, the role of habits cannot be understated. Everything about health boils down to either adding a new habit or cutting down on some old ones. This can be perceived as a stumbling block but can also emerge as a source of enormous strength. For example, I recently decided to inculcate the habit of eating dinner at 5 p.m. and changing an old habit of eating my last meal of the day late at night. I know this sounds off but stay with me for a minute. Once I started looking into my sleep patterns and sleep scores, I noticed that I wasn't getting enough restful sleep despite spending many hours in bed. After much analysis and experimentation, I realized that the culprit was the fact that I'd often eat just an hour or two before my bedtime. When you eat a full meal, your body needs to do vast quantities of work to digest the food and ferry nutrients from the stomach to all parts of the body. While you try to sleep after a meal, the body is actually hard at work, defeating the purpose of getting rest. So, I gradually started moving my dinner time up, but it wasn't easy and I kept falling back into old habits. After several deliberate changes to my environment, such as external reminders and support I was finally able to move my dinnertime up to 5 p.m., and I have dramatically better sleep results to show for it. And no, I have not stopped going out every now and then—I just remember not to wear my Oura Ring on those evenings, so that I'm not sweating when I see the bad scores the next morning.

We have to consider ourselves incredibly lucky to be living in these times. Even the last few decades have made an enormous difference in the science of healthy lifestyles, ranging from nutrition and exercise to meditation and sleep. A lot of pseudoscience has been replaced with real science, with a large amount of peer reviewed research, to back this deep and modern understanding of health. With PET scans and fMRIs, we are able to watch changes in the brain in real-time, to update our understanding of what's working and what's not. Highly accurate wearable devices bring cutting-edge health measurements from hospitals and research labs to people's homes and wrists. Armed with so much knowledge and so many tools, it will be foolhardy to ignore all this and continue to be stuck in outdated ways—unless those outdated ways of life are ones your great-grandparents followed because they evolved from thousands of years of practice and continue to be relevant even today!

We have completed a whirlwind tour of the world of health. It has been an odyssey for humanity in the last 100 years—going from crude measurements of calories and watching musclemen perform for money to unlocking how health really works, knocking on the doors of dramatic life extension and even dabbling with ideas of immortality. While the science of health is complicated, and making habit changes is genuinely hard, what you need to know is really simple. If you remember nothing else from this book, just remembering and practicing the following will do you a world of good!

SLEEP MORE, EAT LESS AND ALWAYS MOVE.

These seven words contain the distilled wisdom of everything we know about a healthy lifestyle. Let the journey of great health begin now!

NOTES

CHAPTER 1

1. Christine Ro, 'The theory of Dunbar's number holds that we can only really maintain about 150 connections at once. But is the rule true in today's world of social media?', *BBC Future* (9 October 2019), https://www.bbc.com/future/article/20191001-dunbars-number-why-we-can-only-maintain-150-relationships.
2. Richard Weindruch and Rajinder S. Sohal, 'Caloric Intake and Ageing', *New England Journal of Medicine* 337 (1997): 986–994.
3. Olivia Solon, 'Ex-Facebook president Sean Parker: site made to exploit human "vulnerability"', *The Guardian* (9 November 2017), https://www.theguardian.com/technology/2017/nov/09/facebook-sean-parker-vulnerability-brain-psychology.
4. A.M. Tsatsakis et al., 'The dose response principle from philosophy to modern toxicology: The impact of ancient

philosophy and medicine in modern toxicology science',
Toxicology Reports, Vol. 5 (2018).

5.   Richard N.W.Wohns, 'Editorial. What doesn't kill you makes
     you stronger', *Journal of Neurosurgery*, Vol. 49: Issue 5 (2020).

6.   Aliya Alimujiang et al., 'Association Between Life Purpose
     and Mortality Among US Adults Older Than 50 Years', *The
     Journal of the American Medical Association Network Open*,
     Vol. 2, no. 5 (May 2019).

7.   Julianne Holt-Lunstad, Timothy B. Smith and J. Bradley
     Layton, 'Social Relationships and Mortality Risk: A Meta-
     analytic Review', *Public Library of Science Medicine*, Vol. 7,
     no. 7 (July 2010).

8.   Nick Cullather, 'The Foreign Policy of the Calorie', *The
     American Historical Review* (2007).

CHAPTER 2

1.   Chin Jou, 'Counting Calories', *Distillations from the Science
     History Institute* (8 April 2011), https://www.sciencehistory.
     org/distillations/counting-calories.

2.   Nick Cullather, 'The Foreign Policy of the Calorie,' *The
     American Historical Review*, Vol. 12, no. 2 (2007).

3.   Christin E. Kearns et al., 'Sugar Industry and Coronary Heart
     Disease Research: A Historical Analysis of Internal Industry
     Documents', *Journal of the American Medical Association—
     Internal Medicine* (November 2016).

4.   Siddhartha Mukherjee, *The Gene: An Intimate History* (Simon
     & Schuster, 2016), p. 21.

5.   Siddhartha Mukherjee, *The Gene: An Intimate History* (Simon
     & Schuster, 2016), p. 25.

6. Siddhartha Mukherjee, *The Gene: An Intimate History* (Simon & Schuster, 2016).

7. T. Colin Campbell and Thomas M. Campbell, *The China Study: The Most Comprehensive Study of Nutrition Ever Conducted and the Startling Implications for Diet, Weight Loss and Long Term Health* (BenBella Books Inc., December 2016).

8. Syed S. Mahmood, Daniel Levy and Thomas J. Wang, 'The Framingham Heart Study and the Epidemiology of Cardiovascular Diseases: A Historical Perspective', *Lancet* (March 2014).

9. Pett KD, Kahn J, Willett WC, Katz DL, 'Ancel Keys and the Seven Countries Study: An Evidence-based Response to Revisionist Histories', *White Paper, True Health Initiative,* (August 2017).

10. 'Apple Heart Study demonstrates ability of wearable technology to detect atrial fibrillation', *Stanford Medicine News Centre* (16 March 2019).

11. Jessica Baron, 'Apple Announced Three New Healthcare Studies And Now Is The Time To Ask Hard Questions', *Forbes* (11 September 2019), https://www.forbes.com/sites/jessicabaron/2019/09/11/apple-announced-three-new-healthcare-studies-and-now-is-the-time-to-ask-hard-questions.

12. Lance D. Dalleck and Len Kravitz, 'The History of Fitness', *The University of New Mexico*, https://www.unm.edu/~lkravitz/Article%20folder/history.html.

13. Grant Christman, 'The Atkins Diet: An Unresolved Debate', *Nutrition Noteworthy*, Vol. 5: 1 (2002).

14. Rachel Link, 'The GM Diet Plan: Lose Fat in Just 7 Days?', *Healthline* (4 July 2017), https://www.healthline.com/nutrition/gm-diet.

15. https://www.statista.com/statistics/617136/digital-population-worldwide/.

16. Gary Taubes, *Good Calories, Bad Calories: Challenging the Conventional Wisdom on Diet, Weight Control, and Disease* (Alfred A. Knopf, New York, 2007).

17. Ingrid G. Farreras, 'History of Mental Illness', General Psychology: Required Reading by Lauren Brewer, *Noba Project* (2019).

CHAPTER 3

1. Michael Pollan, *Food Rules: An Eater's Manual* (Penguin Books, 2009).

2. Christie Nicholson, 'Self-Experimenters: Filmmaker Gained Weight to Prove a Point about Portion Size', *Scientific American* (11 March 2008), https://www.scientificamerican. com/article/filmmaker-gained-weight-to-prove-point/.

3. Dr David Perlmutter and Kristin Loberg, *Grain Brain: The Surprising Truth About Wheat, Carbs and Sugar—Your Brain's Silent Killers* (Little, Brown and Company, 2013).

4. Rosebud Roberts et al., 'Relative Intake of Macronutrients Impacts Risk of Mild Cognitive Impairment or Dementia,' *Journal of Alzheimer's Disease* (2012).

5. Anthony Sclafani and Deleri Springer, 'Dietary Obesity in Adult Rats: Similarities to Hypothalamic and Human Obesity Syndromes', *Physiology and Behavior* (1976).

6. Job Heggie, 'Life is Sweet: The Sugar Story', *National Geographic* (5 February 2019), https://www.nationalgeographic.com/ science/article/partner-content-the-sugar-story.

7. Justin Sonnenburg and Erica Sonnenburg, *The Good Gut: Taking Care of Your Weight, Your Mood and Your Long-Term Health* (Penguin Books, 2015).

8. Richard T. Liu, Rachel F.L. Walsh, Ana E. Sheehan, 'Prebiotics and probiotics for depression and anxiety: A systematic review and meta-analysis of controlled clinical trials', *Neuroscience & Behavioral Reviews* (2019).

9. Stephanie L. Shnorr et al., 'Gut Microbiome of the Hadza Hunter–Gatherers', *Nature Communications* (2014).

10. Philip J. Tuso et al., 'Nutritional Update for Physicians: Plant-Based Diet', *The Permanente Journal* (2013).

11. Deyin Liu et al, 'Calorie Restriction with or without Time-Restricted Eating in Weight Loss', *The New England Journal of Medicine* (2022).

12. A.V. Klein and H. Kiat, 'Detox Diets for Toxin Elimination and Weight Management: A Critical Review of the Evidence', *Journal of Human Nutrition and Dietetics* (2014).

CHAPTER 4

1. Lynne Shallcross, 'Your Chair Is Killing You. Here's What You Need To Do To Stop It', *NPR* (6 October 2015), https://www.npr.org/sections/health-shots/2015/10/06/446295001/your-chair-is-killing-you-here-s-what-you-need-to-do-to-stop-it.

2. Benjamin Baddely, Sangeetaha Sornalingam, Max Cooper, 'Sitting is the new smoking: where do we stand?', *British Journal of General Practice* (May 2016).

3. J.N. Morris et al., 'Coronary Heart-disease and Physical Activity of Work', *Lancet* (1953).

4. Peter Schnohr et al., 'Dose of Jogging and Long-Term Mortality: The Copenhagen City Heart Study', *Journal of the American College of Cardiology* (2015).

5. Cosimo Roberto Russo, 'The Effects of Exercise on Bone. Basic Concepts and the Implications for the Prevention of Fractures', *Clinical Cases in Mineral and Bone Metabolism* (2009).

6. Maria Grazia et al., 'The Effectiveness of Physical Exercise on Bone Density in Osteoporotic Patients', *Biomed Research International* (2018).

7. Simon Melov et al., 'Resistance Exercise Reverses Ageing in Human Skeletal Muscle,' *PLoS One* (2007).

8. Darren G. Candow et al., 'Short-Term Heavy Resistance Training Eliminates Age-Related Deficits In Muscle Mass And Strength In Healthy Older Males', *Journal of Strength and Conditioning Research* (2011).

9. Julia C. Basso and Wendy A. Suzuki, 'The Effects of Acute Exercise on Mood, Cognition, Neurophysiology, and Neurochemical Pathways: A Review', *Brain Plasticity* (2017).

10. James A. Blumenthal et al., 'Exercise and Pharmacotherapy in the Treatment of Major Depressive Disorder', *Psychosomatic Medicine* (2007).

11. Shashi K Agarwal, 'Cardiovascular Benefits of Exercise', *International Journal of General Medicine* (2012).

12. Bente Klarlund Pederson, 'Anti-inflammatory Effects of Exercise: Role in Diabates and Cardiovascular Disease', *European Journal of Clinical Investigation* (2017).

13. Jennifer Scheid and Emma O'Donnell, 'Revisiting Heart Rate Target Zones Through the Lens of Wearable Technology',

American College of Sports Medicine's Health & Fitness Journal (2019).

14. Daniel E. Lieberman, *Why Something We Never Evolved to Do Is Healthy and Rewarding* (Pantheon Books, 2020).

15. Matthew Rhea et al., 'A Meta-Analysis to Determine the Dose Response for Strength Development', *Medicine & Science in Sports & Exercise* (2003).

16. Dr Andrew Huberman, interview with Dr Duncan French, 8 November 2021, in Huberman Lab Podcast #45, https:// podcastnotes.org/huberman-lab/episode-45-dr-duncan-french-how-to-exercise-for-optimal-strength-gains-hormone-optimization-huberman-lab/.

17. Corinne Mulley, Klaus Gebel & Ding Ding, *Walking: Connecting Sustainable Transport with Health* (Emerald Publishing, 2017).

18. Susan Beckham and Michael Harper, 'Functional Training: Fad or Here to Stay?', *American College of Sports Medicine's Health and Fitness Journal* (2010).

19. P. Nolan et al., 'The Effect of Detraining after a Period of Training on Cardiometabolic Health in Previously Sedentary Individuals', *International Journal of Environmental Research and Public Health* (2018).

20. Tom F. Cuddy, 'Reduced Exertion High-Intensity Interval Training is More Effective at Improving Cardiorespiratory Fitness and Cardiometabolic Health than Traditional Moderate-Intensity Continuous Training', *International Journal of Environmental Research and Public Health* (2019).

21. Tiffany Field, 'Yoga Clinical Research Review', *Complementary Therapies in Clinical Practice* (2011).

22. Roger Jahnke et al., 'A Comprehensive Review of Health Benefits of Qigong and Tai Chi', *American Journal of Health Promotion* (2010).

23. Abigail Zuger, 'Too Little Fat Can Be As Bad As Too Much', *The New York Times* (6 July 2004), https://www.nytimes.com/2004/07/06/health/too-little-fat-can-be-as-bad-as-too-much.html?_r=0

24. Dr Andrew Huberman, 'Science of Muscle Growth, Increasing Strength and Muscle Recovery', 31 May 2021, Huberman Labs Podcast #22, https://hubermanlab.com/science-of-muscle-growth-increasing-strength-and-muscular-recovery/ .

CHAPTER 5

1. Shahrad Taheri et al., 'Short Sleep Duration Is Associated with Reduced Leptin, Elevated Ghrelin, and Increased Body Mass Index', *PLOS Medicine* (December 2004).

2. Stephanie Greer, Matthew Walker and Andrea Goldstein, 'The Impact of Sleep Deprivation on Food Desire in the Human Brain', *Nature Communications* (August 2013).

3. Sumathi Reddy, 'How Sleep Has Changed in the Pandemic: Insomnia, Late Bedtimes, Weird Dreams', *The Wall Street Journal* (1 June 2020), https://www.wsj.com/articles/how-sleep-has-changed-in-the-pandemic-insomnia-late-bedtimes-weird-dreams-11591022182.

4. R.K. Dishman et al., 'Decline in cardiorespiratory fitness and odds of sleep complaints', *Medicine and Science in Sports and Exercise* (2015).

5. Kelly Glazer Baron, Kathryn J. Reid and Phyllis C. Zee, 'Exercise to Improve Sleep in Insomnia: Exploration of the Bidirectional Effects', *Journal of Clinical Sleep Medicine* (2013).

6. Irshaad O. Ebrahim, Colin M. Shapiro, Adrian J. Williams and Peter B. Fenwick, 'Alcohol and Sleep I: Effects on Normal Sleep,' *Alcoholism, Clinical and Experimental Research*, Vol 37, no. 4: 539–549.

7. Arianna Huffington, *The Sleep Revolution: Transforming Your Life, One Night at a Time* (Harmony Books, 2016), p. 195.

8. Jason C. Ong, Shauna L. Shapiro and Rachel Manber, 'Mindfulness Meditation and Cognitive Behavioral Therapy for Insomnia: Naturalistic 12-Month Follow-Up', *Explore: The Journal of Science & Healing*, Vol. 5, Issue 1 (2009): 30--36.

9. Matthew Walker, *Why We Sleep: Unlocking the Power of Sleep and Dreams* (Penguin, 2018), p. 164.

10. Matthew Walker, *Why We Sleep: Unlocking The Power of Sleep and Dreams* (Penguin, 2018), p. 173.

11. Aric A. Prather, Denise Janicki-Deverts, Martica H. Hall and Sheldon Cohen, 'Behaviorally Assessed Sleep and Susceptibility to the Common Cold', *Sleep* (2015).

12. Derk-Jan Dijk et al., 'Effects of insufficient sleep on circadian rhythmicity and expression amplitude of the human blood transcriptome', *Proceedings of the National Academy of Science of the USA* (2013).

13. W. Chris Winter, *The Sleep Solution: Why Your Sleep is Broken and How to Fix It* (New American Library, 2017), p. 201.

14. Brice Faraut et al., 'Napping reverses the salivary interleukin-6 and urinary norepinephrine changes induced by sleep restriction', *Journal of Clinical Endocrinology and Metabolism* (2015).

15. Junxin Li et al., 'Afternoon napping and cognition in Chinese older adults: Findings from the China Health and Retirement

Longitudinal Study Baseline Assessment', *Journal of the American Geriatrics Society* (2016).

CHAPTER 6

1. Jean-William Fitting, 'From Breath to Respiration', *Respiration* (2015).
2. James Nestor, *Breath: The New Science of a Lost Art* (Penguin Random House, 2020).
3. George Catlin, *Shut Your Mouth and Save Your Life* (1870), https://buteykoclinic.com/wp-content/uploads/2019/04/Shut-your-mouth-Catlin.pdf.
4. James Nestor, *Breath: The New Science of a Lost Art* (Riverhead Books, New York, 2020).
5. John Douillard, 'The Science Behind Why Nose Breathing Is Better', *LifeSpa* (20 November 2014), https://lifespa.com/finally-research-nose-breathing-exercise/.
6. Ranil Jayawardena et al., 'Exploring the Therapeutic Benefits of Pranayama (yogic breathing): A systematic Review', *International Journal of Yoga* (2020).
7. Ashley Ross, 'How Meditation Went Mainstream', *TIME*, (9 March 2016), https://time.com/4246928/meditation-history-buddhism/.
8. Kieran C. R. Fox, 'Is Meditation Associated with Altered Brain Structure? A Systematic Review and Meta-Analysis of Morphometric Neuroimaging in Meditation Practitioners', *Neuroscience and Biobehavioural Reviews* (2014).
9. Eileen Luders et al., 'Estimating Brain Age Using High-Resolution Pattern Recognition: Younger Brains in Long-Term Meditation Practitioners', *NeuroImage* (2016).

CHAPTER 7

1. Jason Fung, *The Obesity Code: Unlocking the Secrets of Weight Loss* (Greystone Books, 2015), p. 70.
2. Jason Fung, *The Obesity Code: Unlocking the Secrets of Weight Loss* (Greystone Books, 2015), p. 86.
3. Gary Taubes, *Why We Get Fat And What to Do About It* (Anchor Books, 2011), p. 99.
4. Sylvia Tara, *The Secret Life of Fat: The Science Behind the Body's Least Understood Organ and What it Means for You* (W.W. Norton & Company, 2016), p. 2.
5. Sylvia Tara, *The Secret Life of Fat: The Science Behind the Body's Least Understood Organ and What it Means for You* (W.W. Norton & Company, 2016), p. 2.

CHAPTER 8

1. Kasper Hoebe, Edith Janssen and Bruce Beutler, 'The interface between innate and adaptive immunity', *Nature Immunology* (2004).
2. Mary Payne Bennett and Cecile Lengacher, 'Humor and Laughter May Influence Health IV. Humor and Immune Function', *Evidence-Based Complementary and Alternative Medicine* (2009).
3. Matt Richtel, *An Elegant Defense: The Extraordinary New Science of the Immune System* (Mariner Books, 2019), p. 74.
4. See https://norkinvirology.wordpress.com/2015/05/20/felix-dherelle-the-discovery-of-bacteriophages-and-phage-therapy/.

5. Edward Yu et al., 'Diet, Lifestyle, Biomarkers, Genetic Factors, and Risk of Cardiovascular Disease in the Nurses' Health Studies', *American Journal of Public Health* (2016).
6. Janett Barbaresko, Johanna Rienks and Ute Nothlings, 'Lifestyle Indices and Cardiovascular Disease Risk: A Meta-Analysis', *American Journal of Preventive Medicine* (2018).

CHAPTER 9

1. Kavitha Kolappa, David C. Henderson and Sandeep P. Kishore, 'No physical health without mental health: Lessons unlearned?', *Bulletin of the World Health Organization* 91, no. 1 (1 January 2013).
2. Thomas Hobbes, *Leviathan or The Matter, Forme and Power of a Commonwealth, Ecclesasticall and Civil* (Cambridge University Press, 1904).
3. Bessel Van Der Kolk, *The Body Keeps the Score: Brain, Mind, and Body in the Healing of Trauma* (Penguin, 2014).
4. 'Social isolation, loneliness in older people pose health risks', National Institute on Aging—Featured Research, (23 April 2019).
5. Ruta Clair et al., 'The effects of social isolation on wellbeing and life satisfaction during pandemic', *Humanities and Social Sciences Communication* (27 January 2021).
6. Giada Pietrebissa and Susan G. Simpson, 'Psychological Consequences of Social Isolation During COVID-19 Outbreak', *Frontiers in Psychology* (9 September 2020).
7. 'Japan appoints Minister of Loneliness to tackle suicide rates', *Business Today* (24 February 2021), https://www.businesstoday. in/latest/world/story/japan-appoints-loneliness-minister-to-tackle-suicide-rates-289247-2021-02-24.

8. Gururaj G. et al., 'National Mental Health Survey of India, 2015-6: Summary'. Bengaluru, National Institute of Mental Health and Neuro Sciences, NIMHANS Publication No. 130 (2016).

CHAPTER 10

1. Anonymous, *The Homeric Hymns and Homerica with an English Translation by Hugh G. Evelyn-White. Homeric Hymns* (Cambridge, MA., Harvard University Press; London, William Heinemann Ltd.,1914).
2. Daniel J. Levitin, *Successful Ageing: A Neuroscientist Explores the Power and Potential of Our Lives* (Canada: Dutton, 2020), p. 195.
3. Elissa S. Epel, Elizabeth H. Blackburn et al., 'Accelerated telomere shortening in response to life stress', *Proceedings of the National Academy of Sciences of the USA* 101 (49) (December, 2004): 17312-15.
4. J.E. Verhoeven et al., 'Anxiety Disorders and Accelerated Cellular Ageing', *British Journal of Psychiatry* 206 (5) (May, 2015): 371-378.
5. L.F. Cherkas et al., 'The Association Between Physical Activity in Leisure Time and Leukocyte Telomere Length', *Archives of Internal Medicine* 168 (2) (January 2008):154-8.
6. Lee Know, *Mitochondria and the Future of Medicine: The Key to Understanding Disease, Chronic Illness, Aging and Life Itself* (Vermont, USA: Chelsea Green Publishing, 2018), p. 134.
7. Dan Buettner, *The Blue Zones: 9 Lessons for Living Longer from the People Who've Lived the Longest, National Geographic* (2008).

8. Dan Buettner, *The Blue Zones: 9 Lessons for Living Longer from People Who've Lived the Longest* (National Geographic, 2008), p. 83.
9. Denise C. Park et al., 'The Impact of Sustained Engagement on Cognitive Function in Older Adults: The Synapse Project', *Psychological Science* 25 (1) (2013): 103–112.

CHAPTER 11

1. Bertrand Russell, *Portraits from Memory and Other Essays* (Gardeners Books, 1995).
2. Craig R. Whitney, 'Jeanne Calment, World's Elder, Dies at 122,' *The New York Times* (5 August 1997), https://www.nytimes.com/1997/08/05/world/jeanne-calment-world-s-elder-dies-at-122.html.
3. Elisabetta Barbi et al., 'The plateau of human mortality: Demography of longevity pioneers,' *Science* 360 (6396): 1459–61.
4. Chris Neale et al., 'Cognitive effects of two nutraceuticals Ginseng and Bacopa benchmarked against modafinil: a review and comparison of effect sizes', *British Journal of Clinical Pharmacology* 75 (3) (2013): 728–737.
5. Scott Carney, *The Wedge: Evolution, Consciousness, Stress and the Key to Human Resilience* (USA: Foxtopus Ink, 2020), p. 31.